Surviving Brain Injury:
Stories of Strength and Inspiration

Surviving Brain Injury:
Stories of Strength and Inspiration

Compiled by Amy Zellmer
Award-winning author of
Life With a Traumatic Brain Injury: Finding the Road Back to Normal

Surviving Brain Injury: Stories of Strength and Inspiration
©Copyright 2016 by Amy Zellmer.

All rights reserved

No part of this book may be reproduced in any form whatsoever, by photography or xerography or by any other means, by broadcast or transmission, by translation into any kind of language, nor by recording electronically or otherwise, without permission in writing from the author, except by a reviewer, who may quote brief passages in critical articles or reviews.

First Printing 2016

20 19 18 17 16   5 4 3 2 1

Published by Amy Zellmer, Saint Paul, Minnesota
Edited by Connie Anderson, Words & Deeds, Inc.
Cover photo and design by Amy Zellmer
Printing by FuzionPrint

Surviving Brain Injury: Stories of Strength and Inspiration is a work of nonfiction. The names, details, and circumstances may have been changed to protect the survivor's identity.

Dedicated to Tina…

you were taken from this world far too soon, but I feel your presence with me every single day. I know you would be incredibly proud of this book and the advocacy work that I am doing for brain injury awareness.

Table of Contents

Foreword xi
Acknowledgments xii
Thank you to our supporters xiii
Introduction xv
10 Ways You Can Help a Loved One Cope With Their Brain Injury
   Amy Zellmer xvii

1. I'm Still Aaron! — *Aaron Grossman* 1
2. Stronger Than My Struggle — *Adrienne Monroe* 3
3. Life Lessons Learned — *Alice England* 7
4. My Life Has Come Full Circle – *Alyson Ankrom* 12
5. The Gifts of mTBI – *Amiee M. Duffy* 15
6. All We Need Is Just a Little Patience – *Amy Hastings* 18
7. On a Dime – *Amy London* 22
8. Noggin Nonsense: The Harder the Hit …. – *Amy Pilotte* 28
9. Finding the Right Treatment and Doctors Has Been a 19-Year Struggle – *Anne Forest* 31
10. The Best Thing About Miracles Is That They Happen – *Austin Clayton Craft* 37
11. Brought to My Knees – *Barbara Myers* 39
12. How Women Respond and React Differently to Injuries: Specifically Brain Injuries — *Dr. Beth Westie* 44
13. Blessed by a Brain Tumor — *Brenda L. Kleinsasser* 48
14. If This Is Lucky, I Fold — *Carissa Nielsen* 52
15. I May Look Fine, But I'm Not - *Carol Yost* 56
16. Sharing Hard-Earned Advice — *Caroline Charpentier* 61
17. The Day I Chose Life — *Cat Castellanos* 64
18. One Woman, One Trike, 5,390 Miles — *Catherine Brubaker* 67

19. Surviving and Thriving — *Cathy Stewart* 70
20. Always a Driven Person — *Christelle Kay Harris* 72
21. Taking Control of My New Normal — *Courtney G. Lee* 76
22. A Second Can Change Your Life Forever — *Cyndi Syverson* 81
23. C'est la Vie — *Danielle Houston Karst* 84
24. Beyond Survival — *Darcy L. Keith* 89
25. Adopting a Never-Give-Up Attitude — *David Rowlands* 94
26. I Will Fly With Broken Wings — *Deep* 98
27. The Magic of Music — *Derek A. O'Neal* 104
28. The Day That Changed Everything — *Diane Keyes* 110
29. Nightmare in the TBI Disability Lane — *Donna O'Donnell Figurski* 114
30. My First TBI Lesson: When "Alone" Becomes "Lonely" — *Elizabeth Keene Alton* 120
31. I'm Fine — *Ellen Shaughnessy* 125
32. Live Life Large — *Emma Glover* 127
33. Struck Down, But Not Destroyed — *Eryn Adle* 132
34. Almost Dying Saved My Life — *James Manning* 136
35. I Hate What Happened To You--But It Was Bound To Happen — *Jane M* 140
36. Road Bicyclist--Wear a Helmet — *Jeff Squires* 144
37. Take a Walk in My Shoes — *Jennifer Reaid Goodman* 147
38. Helping Others Through Experience — *Dr. Jeremy Schmoe* 150
39. My Feisty Little Brain — *Jessica McCarthy* 154
40. You Are Not Alone — *Joanne Ritchey* 159
41. I Had Always Hoped — *Jocelyn Schwartz* 165
42. Injured Cop Survives Brain Injury — *Jon R. Casey* 167
43. One Careless Driver Changed My Life's Trajectory — *Julia Potocnjak-Overn* 174

44. I'm a "Recovery In Progress" — *Juliette Fiechtner* 178
45. My Son Ryan — *Kathleen Whidden* 181
46. The Lady "Bug" Begins to Fly — *Kathryn Duffy* 183
47. Seeing Brain Rages First Hand — *Dr. Kevin Morford* 188
48. Broken-Hearted Mom — *Kimilie Drew* 193
49. Dear Survivor — *Krystal Decker* 194
50. An Unexpected Four-Legged Friend from the Darkness — *Kurt Trahan* 197
51. What I can Remember — *Lee Staniland* 203
52. A Tumor the Size of a Walnut — *Lisa Cohen* 207
53. Living My New Life — *Louisa Reid* 209
54. Invisible Injuries Can be the Hardest to Diagnose … and to Heal — *Lynn Julian* 213
55. From Victim to Survivor — *Makenzie Biggs* 222
56. The Unfortunate Slip — *Mary Frasier* 226
57. Body Painting: A Caged Mind — *May Mutter* 230
58. Our Post-TBI Honeymoon — *Melissa Jirovec* 233
59. Not By Accident — *Michael Ray Music* 236
60. "No Boundaries" Anymore — *Molly Raymond* 241
61. TBI: To Become Invincible — *Nick Dennen* 245
62. Pushing Past Fear — *Nikki Abramson* 249
63. Dakota Strong — *Nita Massey* 253
64. The Gift of a Near-Fatal Fall — *Pamela Leigh Richards* 255
65. In a Blink of An Eye: Life After Brain Injury — *Paul Bosworth* 261
66. Waiting for the Silver Lining — *Rebecca Hannam* 267
67. I Am a Fighter — *Renie Bania* 271
68. Our Recovery Never Stops — *Ric Johnson* 273
69. An Incredibly Unexpected New Direction — *Rick Smith* 277

70. The Concussion That Changed My Life — *Robert Lee* 280
71. My Life's Journey — *Robyn Alexander* 284
72. Expect Miracles — *Robyn Block* 287
73. My Many Miracles — *Sarana Spokes* 290
74. The Invisible Years — *Sera Rathbun* 295
75. Our Story of Poisoning — and of Grace — *Shelley Taylor and Taylor Trammell* 299
76. From a Dream to a Nightmare to Reality — *Shelly Lorden* 303
77. I'm Very Grateful — *Shelly Millsap* 307
78. Life Is A Lesson — *Stanley H. Wotring, Jr.* 311
79. The Power of Never Giving Up — *Stephanie M. Freeman* 314
80. Post-Traumatic Stress Disorder and Traumatic Brain Injury — USMC — *Stevena Pen* 316
81. Medical Resident Finds a New Life After Suffering Terrible Stroke — *Summer Blackhurst* 318
82. The Way the Wind Blows — *Susan Cason Blackburn* 321
83. Fighting Through It All — *Tammy A. Martin* 323
84. Walk, Bang, Knockout — *Tania Topping* 327
85. My TBI: Moment-by-Moment — *Ted Morin* 333
86. Ten Things I Learned to Help Someone With a TBI — *Toni Popkin* 341
87. Finding My New Normal — *Wendy Squire* 346

Resources 351
International Resources 352
Meet the Models 353
About the Author 356

Foreword

I became "an unwilling expert" as I watched my husband go from a happy, loving man to a dark shadow of his former self. Grant played center in the NFL for 117 games, most of those for the Seattle Seahawks. The skull-battering, jaw-shaking collisions he absorbed during those years ultimately caused him to have numerous concussions. Our life together became a living hell as Grant chose alcohol to medicate for a disease rooted in the scores of concussions he suffered on the football field. This destroyed our marriage of 29 years, and fractured our family.

Grant died on July 15, 2012, at the age of 52, the victim of alcohol abuse and a degenerative brain disease known as chronic traumatic encephalopathy, or CTE.

I now know more about traumatic brain injuries than I ever wanted to know—and I am committed to raising awareness of CTE and the dangers of repetitive head injury.

I applaud Amy Zellmer's effort to bring together so many people who have shared their very personal and sometimes heart-breaking stories—but all 90 of them are a step forward, as telling their stories will help to make others more aware of the seriousness of this invisible injury.

I related so well to a statement in one of the stories: Why don't we have the same empathy, patience and understanding for those with brain injuries as we do for those who have other invisible diseases like heart attack or cancer?

Together we have to work to make brain injuries "more visible" to the public and family members and friends in order to bring these suffering people more understanding, patience, and compassion.

— Cyndy Feasel
Former NFL wife and author of *After the Cheering Stops: An NFL Wife's Story of Concussions, Loss, and the Faith That Saw Her Through*
www.afterthecheeringstops.com

Acknowledgments

This book was truly a community project, and I thank each and every contributor who participated. With this book we will continue to raise awareness of this invisible injury across the globe.

For all who backed this book on Kickstarter and helped make it a reality, I thank you on behalf of everyone involved. For many, this is the first time they have shared their story.

To the Tribe for your continued support and encouragement. You all truly inspire me in ways that words cannot describe.

To Jill, for you always have brilliant ideas—no matter how crazy they seem at the time.

To Simon, for your countless hours of moral support—and sushi.

To Connie, for your patience and compassion during the editing phase, and for not freaking out on my crazy deadline.

To all of the amazing women in my writing group, and especially Ann, Sherri, Meg, Cathy, and Colleen, each and every one of you has touched me in profound ways.

To Katlyn, for being a shiny reminder of how much I love all things pink and glittery.

To Bruce, for your DJ skills and willingness to always come to my rescue.

To Dr. Jeremy Schmoe and everyone at MFNC Brain Rehabilitation, for truly understanding me and helping me get the rehab that I need.

Thank you to our supporters

Alan and Jane Glover

Amy M. Pilotte

Andrew D. and Tara J. Filicicchia

Brain Injury Services of Virginia

Caroline Brethenoux

Cashelle Dunn

Catherine Brubaker M.S.L., Executive Director Hope For Trauma

D. Chadwick Hurst

Emma Glover

Erynn Adle

Heather Adle

Jack and Patty Dennen

Jan Saddy

Jean Chappell

Joanne Ritchey

John and Alice Hanlon

Kimberly Jones

Olivia Bridewell

Steve Power

Ted Morin

Terry Meehan

Timothy W. Donovan

Walter Krause

Introduction

"You must be the change you wish to see in the world." – Gandhi

This book is truly a community project, a work of art, a piece of magic. It is part of a vision to raise awareness about this invisible injury that affects someone in the United States every 13 seconds—that's 2.5 million Americans annually. Brain injury does not discriminate, and affects every race, income level, nationality, and gender.

This global epidemic is misunderstood and undiagnosed far too often. As you read through the stories, you will catch a glimpse into the many lives that have been changed forever as the result of a brain injury.

If you are a survivor, you will understand the *all-too-familiar chaos* that follows. If you are a loved one, friend, co-worker, or casual friend of someone who has sustained a brain injury, I applaud you for reading this book. It is important you know that what we are going through is very real and very debilitating. Yes, we desperately want you to understand our daily struggles with memory loss, aphasia (not being able to recall words), cognitive deficits, coordination, balance and dizziness issues, headaches, depression and anxiety, unemployment, overstimulation, and so much more. We are in this for the long haul, as it can take months or years to recover—and some of us may never make a full and complete recovery.

This book is not only a tool to bring awareness to the world, it is also a conduit for healing. The contributors have shared their most intimate story—some for the very first time. Telling our story can be incredibly therapeutic, a powerful release of the emotions and baggage that we have bottled up inside.

On the pages that follow, I share an article I originally wrote for *The Huffington Post*, "10 Ways You Can Help a Loved One Cope With Their Brain Injury." I included this as a resource for anyone who isn't sure how to help a friend or loved one through this difficult time.

Keep in mind that while *we may seem fine*, we are going to be recovering for a long time, and we will appreciate acts of kindness at any point in our recovery.

My personal mission is to bring a greater awareness to brain injury, not only to the general public, but also to all medical professionals. Change really can start with just one person, and I have recruited almost 90 others who have willingly shared their stories.

10 Ways You Can Help a Loved One Cope With Their Brain Injury

Amy Zellmer

(Updated from original as published on *The Huffington Post*)

In a recent conversation with my fellow brain injury survivors, we were discussing ways that people can reach out and help us. The first few months after a concussion or brain injury are critical. I know that when I look back at my first six months, I can see how completely dazed and confused I was.

However, the recovery time from a brain injury can from last months to years. Every single brain injury is unique, and will not only take different recovery times, but will also present different symptoms, depending on where the brain was injured.

A brain injury is much like a fingerprint or snowflake—no two are alike.

In addition, many "outsiders" have no idea what kind of hell we are going through. They hear the word "concussion" and think it's not big deal. Or they hear the term "traumatic brain injury," and can only imagine the most severe (think coma, bedridden, not able to speak or walk), and figure if we're walking and talking, then we must be doing "OK." Neither of these scenarios is correct.

I beg you to try to understand what we're going through. At the very least, I offer you some suggestions on how to help us cope with this stressful and frustrating time of our life.

1. Don't ask us what we need. We may not actually know "what" we need. Or we may feel embarrassed and don't want to be a burden or seem needy. Don't ask us if we'd like you to come over. We'll probably say no, but really mean yes. Just show up at our door with open arms. Bring over a meal (or three). We are likely suffering from a great deal of fatigue, headaches, and cognitive problems. We might not have the ability to cook for ourselves, or even go to the grocery store to buy the bare necessities. I could not even figure out how to use my microwave or oven for several days. A warm, home-cooked meal would have been greatly appreciated.

2. Bring us groceries or basic household supplies. As much as we won't admit it, our finances are going to be really, really tight. Going to the grocery store may actually be a financial burden as much as it is a physical one. No one wants to admit when she is struggling, and just showing up with some milk, toilet paper, and chocolate chip cookies will definitely bring joy and relief.

3. Offer to clean our house. Many of us suffer with vertigo, fatigue, and often have physical injuries from our accident. Simple tasks like taking out the garbage, doing laundry, and vacuuming can be daunting. Don't judge the condition of our home, and don't make us feel like we are doing a poor job of housekeeping, simply enter our home and start doing it for us. Take it a step further, and make us a glass of ice water, tuck us into bed for a nap, and clean away while we rest!

4. Offer to drive us to our doctor appointments. I was fortunate that I was able to drive after my accident, but many are not. I also encourage you to go one step further, and ask if we'd like you to sit in on the appointment. I went to all my appointments alone, and as I look back, I realize how little I remember. It would have been nice to have someone along to help advocate for my health, and to be able to explain to the doctor what he or she was observing of my daily behavior, and how it may be altered from my "normal."

5. Get us out of the house. Before you kidnap your loved one or friend, and take her on an adventure, make sure you ask her if she is feeling up to it. If it is an adventure that comes with some monetary costs, make it clear that you are buying (remember that our finances may be really, really tight). Keep in mind that we may be sensitive to light, sounds, crowds, etc. and plan something accordingly. A trip to a flower garden (remind us to bring our sunglasses), or to a spa for a pedicure might be lovely options. You can ask us what we'd like to do, but be prepared for us to not be able to articulate a clear plan. Be prepared to plan it all out.

6. Bring us flowers. I know that's totally cliché, but beautiful flowers can really brighten up anyone's day!

7. Send a card or care package. If you don't live nearby, sending a card stating that you're thinking of us will mean so very much. Just knowing that someone has her thoughts on you can go a long way in recovery. If you're feeling generous, you may also include a gift card to a local grocery or Target store. Also, be sure to check out Healing Boxes, designed specifically for brain injury survivors: www.healing-boxes.com/tbi

8. Show up with a movie and a book. Ask us if we would prefer to watch a movie, or have you read to us. Everyone's TBI is going to be different. Some of us can't handle watching a movie or hearing the sounds, and many can't read well. So offering to read a book to us might really make our day. If neither seem appealing to us at the time, snuggle up with us on the couch under a comfy blanket, and just be there for us. Sometimes sitting in silence with a loved one can really make a person's day.

9. Watch our kids for a few hours. Or better yet, take them overnight. Being a parent with TBI has got to be overwhelming and exhausting. Knowing that our child(ren) is in good hands will give us comfort and allow us to rest and recharge for a few hours. Rest is SO important in the recovery process.

10. Also know that we are in this for the long haul. We will still be struggling with the lasting effects of our injury for months, if not years, after the accident. Don't put pressure on your loved one that we "should" be feeling better. I am over two years out and still suffer a great deal of fatigue as well as dizziness and balance issues

Also know that we tend to be incredibly emotional after a head injury, or possibly even aggressive. Be prepared that your generosity will elicit many emotions, some will cry, some will laugh, and some might possibly get angry with you. Don't take any of it personally we are dealing with a very difficult injury, not to mention a complete change in our personality. Just know that you are doing the best you can for us and that we appreciate you no matter how we may react.

Chapter One
I'm Still Aaron!

Aaron Grossman
Boca Raton, Florida

Well, where to start? Let's see, like most of my fellow survivors, I was sure that I had a whole world ahead of me. I had just graduated college, landed a good-paying, respectable teaching job I was proud of. I had a brand-new car, a girlfriend, and an active social life, with friends, going to events, etc. And I was immortal. What could go wrong?

My stepmom always told me that she hated driving with me because, "One day you're going to get into an accident with the way you jump red lights." Jumping a red light is when a driver proceeds forward when he can see the crossing traffic's light turn red, not waiting for your light to turn green. What did she know? Again, I was unstoppable.

I had just sold the motorcycle I drove all through college and bought a car, you know, to be safer. The 1999 Honda Civic was a very small, lightweight car, like a box of plastic. It certainly was no match for the big metal Lincoln Towncar that hit my driver's side door, spinning my car around, causing me to then get hit by a second car. The airbag deployed, and my jerking into my seatbelt made my body and head shake around violently, giving me a subdural hematoma. The doctors likened it to shaken-baby syndrome. Oh well.

My parents tell me that I was thrust into an immediate coma from the impact, but what was almost my downfall was when I got sick while in the coma. I contracted a staph infection called MRSA, and this pushed me into an even-deeper coma, where I stayed just shy of two months.

Upon waking up, I had no idea where I was, or what had happened. My father and mother were both there, so I had no clue what was different. I only knew that I was disappointed when they left every night, and I never went with them. Why was I even here?

My memory of these few months are very shaky. I do, however, remember finally being able to leave the hospital and go home with my parents, my dad and stepmom Stacey, who I soon started calling Mom. We had three dogs in the house, my parents' small dog, and the two dogs I had in college. Why did I get the dogs instead of one of my four roommates? Oh well.

I started my outpatient rehab; then my vocational rehab. It was only about two years, but it felt like ten years of rehab. They helped me land a job as an assistant at an after-school program for children with various disabilities. I loved what I was doing because I really related to the kids. I really took them home every night with me, in thought. It probably wasn't so smart putting me in charge of a classroom of students with various handicaps, especially so soon after my own accident.

One day, at an outing, two of my children wandered off while I was in charge of looking after them. My boss, a very nice woman, had no choice but to let me go. I don't blame her, of course. My parents couldn't leave me in the house alone while they worked, so Stacey would take me along to her job at a jewelry store in a big shopping mall, five days a week. As one could imagine, that got old very fast for me.

Time has passed since then, I've been working part time as a cashier at an art store for the past ten years. It's pretty mindless stuff, but it is exhaustingly busy. Yes, I'm lonely, and yes, I do want more for my life. I do, though, believe that I'm special, not just lucky. I don't want to waste any more time, I want to start living my life to the fullest, and to stop *just letting life happen*.

Life is hard for *everybody*, we all have hurdles to jump over, some of us, though, just need a little more help and a little more time getting over them because post-TBI laziness is a tall mountain to jump over.

No bio provided.

Chapter Two
Stronger Than My Struggle

Adrienne Monroe
Fort Ashby, West Virginia

I think it's been five years since my car accident (2011), and I am just now feeling like I am somewhat "getting it together." I am not the person I was pre-accident, but I know I never will be. That girl is gone, although sometimes I still find myself trying to find her.

The "new me!" Have you heard that before? I could never figure out what "the new me" meant, and honestly I cannot stand it when I hear someone refer to the newly brain injured person that way. The "new me" makes me think of improvement, of something better. Sorry, but that's not how I feel or think about TBI.

I lost my executive functions, multi-tasking, time management, and short-term memory—the things I excelled at, the things I listed first on my resume. I have issues making decisions. The smallest of choices can still bring me to tears. Pre-TBI, I always said: how do you expect anyone else to like you if you don't like yourself first. I really liked who I was, my drive, determination, goals, and my attitude. All those things seem to have been taken away from me, and I don't think I will ever get that back. In fact, I know I will not get it back.

My doctor says my starter switch was broken in the accident, the process my brain uses to initiate tasks just doesn't seem to work, so I have medication to get it started. It's not the same, but it helps, which is in itself is frustrating. There are things I want and need to do, but just can't seem to do them.

I am a wife and a mother of two, a 14-year-old who is starting high school, and a three-year-old. Yes, he was conceived after my accident. When I first got pregnant, someone asked me: why would you do that with all the issues you have? I asked myself the same thing, but I needed him. I needed him to remind me to get my ass out of bed and to move forward, and stop dwelling on things that cannot change. Plus he remembers where things are, so I can ask him where my phone is, and usually he can find it.

The hardest thing is that no one really understands, they say they try, but they don't have to live in my world. I have to live in theirs.

I need downtime, and for a mother of two who works full time—that is almost impossible to achieve, so more times than not, I am exhausted. I have incorporated strategies, like making a menu for the month so I don't have to think about what to make for dinner, and besides, it's easier to make a grocery list. I have a dry-erase board, so when we run out of something I can write it down right away so I don't forget to put it on my list. I tried to organize my pantry with nice see-through containers so one can see what's in it, but honestly, after going to the grocery store, I am spent. So coming home and putting everything in containers and storing it away all nice and tidy is something from a fairytale. It's not going to happen.

I went back to work two weeks after my accident, because like most middle-class families, we lived paycheck to paycheck. I had ADHD, and suffered from depression as a result of the TBI. After thirty-some odd years of never having to deal with such things, how was I supposed to figure it out now? I still haven't figured it all out; I just cope with it.

It took years to get back to a good place at work, and my employer was less than sympathetic about my issues, and made no attempt to understand. If I worked too much or had stimulation overload, I shut down. Sometimes I worked more than forty hours, which made me physically sick with migraines, and I simply could not function. I would cry on my way to work, cry at lunch, cry on my way home, and then come home, drop into bed and simply melt down. It took years and a couple of changes in medication before I finally felt better. I had no idea how to handle or cope with the things I couldn't do or couldn't remember. Years later, I realized I had a stopping point—and had to stop. I don't work more than forty hours in a week, and weekends are time for rest.

My employer recently had me in his office and told me I have made improvements. My attitude and performance are better, my mistakes are fewer, and I seem to have more drive. I looked at him, saying, "You never gave me a chance to figure things out after my accident. It has taken me this long to get it together. I injured my brain and lost my executive functions. I lost the things that help me do my job well, and I am finally figuring it all out."

My brain is a major organ in my body, so why is it if someone has a heart attack, it's understandable if they are tired and can't do the things they once did. You can't see a heart attack, so how is it that different from a brain injury?

I am not stronger because of my TBI. I was strong before, however I am more humbled, and much more understanding. I long to know who I would be if the person that hit me wasn't in such a hurry, but I think less and less about that as time goes on. Why waste time on something I'll never know.

I have never wanted pity because of my disability. Sometimes I just want to talk about it without someone saying: that happens to me all the time… or, I'm so sorry. Most of the time I simply want some help. I went to therapy for years, and the hardest thing is asking for help. There's always someone saying can you do this or that for me, but no one is asking, "What can I do for you?" Once I hung up the super mom cape, I know that it's okay to keep it off. At this point in my life I am trying to figure out what I want, and what my goals are. I have no idea. So if I can still talk and be understood at the end of the day, and haven't lost my cool, I'm good. Hopefully I will have much more time to figure everything out. I am blessed with a good support system, and a doctor who understands and is truly a godsend in my life.

I still have issues, and I know I always will. I know I will never be who I was, and honestly I don't remember much about her, but I know I will figure it out as I go. I need to continue being stronger than the struggle, and figure it out as I go.

Adrienne Monroe is a brain injury survivor who resides in Fort Ashby, West Virginia, with her husband, Bruce, and two sons.

Chapter Three
Life Lessons Learned

Alice England
Cullman, Alabama

The car accident that caused my TBI happened in April 1996. This year was my twenty-year mark, time goes by so quickly. It's been quite a bumpy ride.

My last vivid memory on the day of the accident was stopping by to see my boyfriend of a few months at the shop where he worked. I had just come from a doctor appointment and was on my way home. James had seemed to be my soul mate from the night we met. We were totally in love, and planned a life together. In fact, in just this short time, I had left my job as a CAD draftsman to become a housewife, my dream job. We were comfortable with only James' salary as a certified auto mechanic, and were deliriously happy with our newfound love.

The accident occurred less than ten minutes later in front of our municipal golf course. I received immediate attention, and was airlifted from the site to the nearest trauma hospital. I have no memory of the accident, but was told that I swerved to miss a dog. I was not wearing my seatbelt—such a stupid, stupid mistake, and *one I will never make again*. When the car flipped, we think that the air bag hit my face, giving me a TBI and the other facial injuries. My injuries included a crushed brow bone, a broken nose, and a tiny cut at the corner of my left eye. I broke my jaw on both sides and broke the roof of my mouth, so my mouth was wired shut for a month. I think I managed to (barely) live through this long, sad month because of both my newfound love…and my strong pain medications.

Lesson 1: Wear your seatbelt.
I was in the NICU for a week and half, but during that time, was always improving. As my mom and James sat and waited for news,

they heard as others were given not-so-good reports, but mine, miraculously were always good, and as you can see, I made it. I had surgery to repair my face, which was done by going under the skin so as to leave no scars. Now I look as if nothing ever happened to me—and, as we survivors of TBI all know, *that's both a blessing and a curse.*

It was a hard first two years. The real me was suddenly gone, before James even got to know me well. I struggled through that time, sleeping for 18 hours many days. Everyone was on edge, and the depression we all experienced was debilitating. In one instance, my mom was at my house helping me, as usual, on a day not long after the accident. Somehow I got mad enough to call the police *to come remove her!* I had never experienced anger like that before. Luckily, the officer was very nice, and he smoothed things over with us and left. My mom was worried by then that my brain was bleeding again, so she finally talked me into going to the local ER. Without going into all the embarrassing details, with my jaw still wired shut, and less than a month post-accident, a young doctor labeled me a drug seeker. I got very defensive and upset, and this time the police were called *on me.* Things that time were also smoothed over, and it was finally determined that the liquid pain medicine I was taking had been stopped too suddenly, causing this bizarre behavior. I was given a last refill to step me down from the high dose, and after this horrible episode, I did fine.

Lesson 2: Your emotions are no longer under your control.

Let me pause to say that without my mom's help, I don't know where I'd be. Through her love and her cheerleading, as well as her persistence to see me to my full recovery, she carried me through all the tough times. She has always loved me unconditionally, and it was vitally important that she still loved the new me—because I am not, and will never be again, the girl she had known all these years. She has not disappointed me at any time.

James was also amazing because he hadn't run for the hills yet. Instead of me serving him breakfast before work as we had imagined, he brought me those instant breakfast drinks before he left for work that I'd then drink through my locked teeth. It was not always pretty, because of all the terrible emotions that were raging—first those of a new relationship, and second, those following a TBI. We were almost sure to fail. James had been married before, and he was my first real boyfriend of my entire life. I was thirty-two then, and was used to living alone with my dog, Einstein, and cat, Tesla.

At first, my mom helped me during the day. It was quite a long time before I even took a shower while alone in the house. My weight plunged to 102 pounds, and I looked like a skeleton in the mirror. To me, the oddest thing about my looks was my pupil variation. I was staring in the mirror one day, literally trying to grasp that I was looking at…myself. Something was grabbing my attention, and I suddenly realized that my pupils were different sizes. When you looked at me, you didn't notice it immediately, but my overall look was of someone slightly dazed and confused, which I was. I was told my brain would retrain the pupils in time, and it did just that. Thank you, my brain…my hero!

Lesson 3: The old me is gone.
I was healing on the outside, and finally the wires were removed from my mouth. As I got better, I began working at a very low-stress job for my cousin, painting decorative furniture with a wonderful group of women in a "paint room" at her store. It was a wonderful time for me, to come or go as I pleased, while still feeling that I was doing something worthwhile. However, I was devastated that after less than a year there, I was feeling too drained to continue. This started an unhappy trend for me. I would stay home, sleep most of the day, and feel like a parasite for as long as I could stand it (a few months usually), then I would feel the need to work again. I took a job at a veterinarian's office, which I loved, but after a while, I again had to resign. I volunteered at a local hospice, and a few years later, at the local mental health center for a few months each, and was hired at both places to work full time. Of course I was thrilled because I loved both jobs, and worked hard at each for about the usual year or so—and then the fatigue that I could never recover from would finally make it impossible for me to continue.

Lesson 4: The fatigue will just about kill you.
After all these tries at regular work, I finally contacted an attorney and filed for disability. Sadly, you will usually need a lawyer. I was

very depressed about all this, the lost jobs and disability issues. In the meantime, James, and my mom, as needed, were still working and caring for me. I had been sputtering like this for about seven years, and I was getting tired of not being any help, as a homemaker or an employed worker—and I was not even receiving disability.

Lesson 5: You normally do not get disability on your own merits.
My disability case had been in the works for nearly two years by now, but it looked as though it was finally to be approved. My gosh, I was so grateful for this help! But almost as soon as the bank deposits began, I received a letter from social services stating that my disability was being re-examined. I was crushed, felling totally helpless and hopeless. So, in February of 2006, I scribbled crazy words on the forms that had been sent to me, put them in the provided envelope and walked them out to my mailbox. I then went back inside and took a whole bottle of Xanax.

Sadly, I was not thinking clearly. My actions meant James would be the one to find me here, and it would cause my pets to feel who knows what kind of anxiety. It still makes me sick to think of my selfishness. I was not successful in my attempt. As I began to get sleepy, I called my mom who called 911, and I was taken to the same trauma center that had saved me from the TBI ten years before. But this time I was on the psychiatric ward, where I was kept for about two weeks until they determined I wouldn't harm myself again. I will never get over the horrible threat I posed to my family that day, of having to go on without me. Nothing on earth is worth your death at your own hand. I am telling you this from my own terrifying experience.

Lesson 6: Please don't ignore feelings of self-harm.
After the suicide attempt, I had to find mental health care services, and I became a patient at the same place I had worked a few years before. At my request, the doctor there gave me something for my severe daytime sleepiness. I began taking Provigil, a drug used for narcolepsy. I realize it is always a good thing to find a natural way to treat medical issues, but this was my last hope after all these years—and it worked! I was staying awake longer, so I was able to get things

done in the house, as per James' and my own dreams at the very beginning. This wakefulness helped my depression in an unbelievable way. I began creating again, and oh my, what a boost that was! I learned to needle felt and began making miniature dogs identical to photographs I received from dog owners all over. I could take my own time, work at home, and meet the most amazing people in this way. Now, I was on my way to recovery of self.

Lesson 7: Things *do* get better!
My life today is my dream. I could not be anywhere doing anything else that would please me more. James and I are still madly in love, most days, and that is the best story I've told here. We have true love, and are soul mates, and work together for a common good. We have five dogs, a cat and a bird that talks. I am still making small felt dogs, and now I also sew doll clothes, a fun thing to do. The person I am today is *me*. I am her, better and wiser and still in this same body, now a little overweight. I have conquered that TBI! And I even love myself again.

One reason for the length of this is due to a problem that remains with me: perseveration, meaning that I go on and on and on. All the paragraphed thoughts I used throughout are a window into the workings of my mind that I wanted to share. If I say one thing, a million other small thoughts carry me away from the subject at hand. Twenty years later, I still suffer from fatigue, and take small naps throughout the day. I go grocery shopping at 7:00 a.m. to avoid the crowd because I get completely confused and usually take forever to make a decision. But I am a survivor of a traumatic brain injury

Lesson 8: Love your *new self!*

Alice is a constant creator, designing gifts for family and friends that are intended to be absolutely perfect. She is madly in love with James, her husband of twenty happy years. They live in a beautiful rural section of central Alabama with five rescue dogs, an amazing cat, and a talking parrot.

Chapter Four
My Life Has Come Full Circle

Alyson Ankrom
Bolivar, Missouri

In 2015, I was an active, healthy mother of four young children, ages 5 and under. As most moms with little ones know, finding enough time for sleeping, eating, exercising, heck, even showering, was a struggle. Of course I was tired and harried. Who wasn't?

Being tired turned into not feeling well...things that had once been done without thought started taking an enormous amount of concentration. Going to the park, once a several-times-a-week activity, just seemed "too hard." I was having difficulty remembering things, or even just listening to my children or my husband. Once a multi-tasking queen, I found myself getting frustrated with seemingly simple tasks; now requiring a calendar and many visual cues to remember what I needed to accomplish. "Get with it, sister!" I'd tell my frustrated self.

My eyesight started to worsen. "Getting older sure stinks!" I thought to myself. Little did I know. As symptoms started to worsen, it prompted a visit to the doctor. An MRI revealed something I don't think anyone ever expects to hear in his or her lifetime: I was officially diagnosed with a brain tumor.

A surgery date was set quickly. Since I was "young" and "healthy" (I always giggle at that because "brain tumor" and "healthy" in the same sentence seemed like such an oxymoron), it was decided that a craniotomy was the best route to resect as much of the tumor as possible. Oh, and since imaging showed that the tumor was directly *in* my motor strip, I'd not only be having my skull opened and part of my brain removed, I'd also be awake while they were doing it. I remember wondering, is this an episode of "Grey's Anatomy" or real life?

I admit, I didn't ask a whole lot of questions about what life would be like post-surgery. I just wanted to get through it. Surprising how a person can change from being a "Google extraordinaire" to hiding under a rock. Ignorance was bliss.

Surgery went well, and I was up and walking the next day, and sent home two days later. I was back to life, back to "normal," except I found out quickly, life wasn't "normal." I was so excited to get back home to my life that I loved so much, only to find out I wasn't quite who I used to be. I couldn't wait to be around the hustle and bustle of my little ones, only I found it was almost unbearable for more than a few minutes at a time. When people asked me questions, it was almost painful. Not the noise (although, it too could be bothersome), but the thinking and processing that went with it. Once I had felt so strong and "tough," now I felt so weak and so bothered. It was overwhelming. In tears I remember wondering if I would ever be me again? And how on earth was I ever going to care for my family (by myself) again?

Going to the grocery store for the first time, I was so overwhelmed that I bought headphones, ripped them out of the package right away so I could listen to music and help block everything else out. Such silly little things that I had never thought about before, were almost like puzzles. I remember writing a thank you card, and couldn't remember how to write the letter b; I wrote a d instead. Thankfully, it didn't last long and I was able to laugh about it. Outings with lots of noise, lights and people had to balance with quiet time. One step forward, two steps back. This was especially frustrating for someone who had always felt like I could "tough it out." It took me a long while to learn *that brain function wasn't a matter of will or fortitude*.

"tough it out" isn't a choice anymore.

As time went on, I improved, even though having radiation treatments, a grand mal seizure, and chemotherapy. I didn't notice it at the time, but as I look back, I realize it was slow and steady. Each week or month I could do a little more. I woke up one day and the sounds of my kids being kids didn't make me want to hide anymore. I didn't have to leave worship services to sit in the back room where the sounds weren't so magnified. I could remove earplugs from my Amazon subscribe and save list. I'm happy to report that just last week, I took all four kids to the park by myself, without a second thought. Something I had thought a year ago was unfathomable, felt like second nature again. It was that day when my life felt full-circle again.

Going through this was hard, and sometimes, it still is. But overall, I am so thankful that our new normal isn't as scary as it once was. There is *always* hope and possibility; just keep taking that one step forward, no matter how daunting it may seem.

Alyson Ankrom is married to her college sweetheart, Darrin, and together they spend their days raising (and chasing!) after their four young children. She loves God, spending time with friends and family, coffee, documenting the little stories of life with photographs, laughing, and healthy doses of sarcasm.

Chapter Five
The Gifts of mTBI

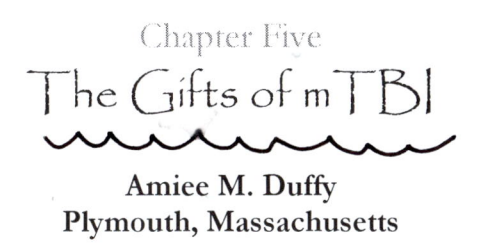

Amiee M. Duffy
Plymouth, Massachusetts

It was a beautiful sunny afternoon at the end of January 2015. I had just picked up my youngest son from school, and was on my way to bring him to his father so I could attend a meeting.

We were driving down a road we had traveled every school day for years. There was no snow, and the roads were dry. Out of the corner of my eye I saw a car that was heading straight toward my driver's side door. I thought, "This doesn't make sense. Where are they coming from?" SLAM!! The car plowed into my driver's side door, and my head bounced off the window.

My hand immediately went to my head, expecting it to be covered in blood. It wasn't. I was dazed and remember feeling like everything was moving in really slow motion, as if I was attempting to walk and talk underwater. I looked in the backseat and asked my nine-year-old if he was okay. Luckily he was seated on the opposite side of the impact, and was wearing his seatbelt.

I tried to get out of the car, but the door was damaged. I was able to crawl over the center console and out of the passenger door into a foot of snow. My Honda Pilot was now in the middle of someone's front lawn. My feet were unsteady and everything was spinning. I felt sick to my stomach as I sat with the door open and my head between my knees.

I could hear people coming while yelling that an ambulance was on its way. I remember trying to not pass out so that my son wouldn't be afraid as I was carried into the back of the ambulance on a backboard in a neck brace. The emergency room was packed and there was no space for me other than in the hallway. The lights, sounds, and smells were overwhelming. I just needed to get out of there and go home! The doctor finally saw me and prescribed some Tylenol and told me I would probably be sore for a few days, but essentially I was fine. My ex-husband arrived to pick up our son and to drive me home. He was the first person to notice. "Amiee, you are not okay. Something is wrong."

I didn't realize it at the time, but I was on my way to learning about traumatic brain injury. As the days went on, I not only had headaches, but I had difficulty speaking. I knew what I wanted to say, but the words either wouldn't come out, or they would come out but I was slurring them or stuttering. Even worse was when I believed I was talking normally and making perfect sense, and my children would look at me and say, "Mom, what are you talking about?"

I had a CAT scan and MRI and everything was "fine." But I WASN'T. I wasn't fine at all. I was sleeping 12–15 hours a day and still not feeling rested. I couldn't communicate with the car insurance company or doctors' offices because I couldn't understand the questions they were asking. I was unable to spontaneously develop questions and ask them in a timely fashion. I was not able to function on my own, and I certainly was unable to take care of my three children. And…when I wasn't sleeping, fear began to creep in.

I was unable to work and originally took just two weeks off. I don't think I truly understood the shape I was in. I began to have issues with short-term memory. I couldn't remember a thing. I wrote down everything I needed to remember, but because I often forgot to look at the sticky notes that were littering my kitchen counter, it didn't really do me any good. I went back to my primary care physician and advocated for me to receive speech and cognitive therapy with a speech and language pathologist.

I went to speech/cognitive therapy three times a week. I struggled to remember three items on a list after a 10-second delay. I could not do third grade math. I still stuttered. My short-term memory was nonexistent. I remained in therapy for six months, a far cry from the original two weeks I thought I would be sidelined.

Over the course of a year I had many appointments—with neurologists, physical therapists, lawyers, and ophthalmologists. I was seen for cognitive delays, executive function problems, memory issues, tinnitus, partial loss of hearing in one ear, sensory issues, anxiety, muscle tension, poor balance, and almost constant migrainous head pain. As I navigated my way through the variety of appointments that year, I had small victories, such as being able to drive to familiar places without having to rely on GPS, and being able to complete grocery shopping without getting sick to my stomach. And finally there were larger victories in that I was able to return to work full time, and also make a five-hour car trip on my own in order to visit my parents.

It has been a year and a half since the motor vehicle accident that changed my life. At times, I still mourn my previous life. So many things changed that I had taken for granted. I wish I had appreciated my body and brain more. I wish I didn't sweat the small stuff as much as I did. However, as with any difficulty that comes slamming into you without warning, there have been gifts.

I am getting better at accepting what is. I rush through life less. I have much more patience with others now. Even better than that, I have much more patience with myself. I am better at giving myself care. I ask for help when I need it. I am getting better at listening to my body. I invest in quality sleep and take time for massages. I make time for activities that bring me joy. I savor the good days when I am pain free. I am using the gift of my mTBI to appreciate all that I have and look forward to continued recovery and promoting awareness.

Amiee M. Duffy is the proud mother of three. She is a public school teacher and a frequent contributor to TBI Hope and Inspiration magazine. Amiee is committed to spreading awareness about mild TBI.

Chapter Six
All We Need Is Just a Little Patience

Amy Hastings
Cold Spring, Kentucky

"Shed a tear, 'cause I'm missin' you. I'm still alright to smile. Girl, I think about you, *every day*, now."

Yes, you read that right. I just quoted the first line of the song, "Patience," by my favorite band of all time, Guns N' Roses. Right about now you're thinking, "Wow! This girl really hit her head…hard." (Well, I did.) Or, if you also have a traumatic brain injury, you might be thinking, "Wow…that's exactly how I feel."

If you've suffered a traumatic brain injury, sooner or later, you come to the realization that the (insert your name here) you used to be is gone, and even though you long to have her back, you know that everything is changed forever. You also eventually realize that you're going to get through this, and something good will come from this tragedy called, traumatic brain injury.

On Wednesday, October 21, 2015 (yes, I know that was also "Back to the Future Day." After all these years, and I missed it!), I took my (then) two-year-old with me to the grocery store. As I was looking for pasta sauce, my vision became blurred, I couldn't focus my eyes, and it felt like my eyes were moving in waves inside my brain. I knew something was very wrong, but strangely, I moved closer to the pasta sauce, still determined to make out the writing on the jar. When I felt a pop in my head, I knew something very bad was about to happen. What, though, I had no idea. I was disoriented, but managed to guide myself back around to the front of the cart, where my daughter was sitting. I dialed my husband's phone number, but he didn't answer.

The next thing I remember is being wheeled down the hallway of a hospital on a gurney, being asked questions that I didn't know the answers to, by people who I did not know.

Based on the two people who witnessed my fall, my description of what happened before I fell, the results of CT scans and other tests, the team of doctors and nurses working to save my life that day, my current doctors, and because there is no benchmark for traumatic brain injuries, this is what we believe may have happened: I had a brain bleed and/or seizure, causing me to pass out and hit my head on the floor, instantly knocking me unconscious. The blow to my head split my head open, also causing numerous broken bones, including the bones around both eye sockets and the back of my skull. After hitting the floor, I suffered a second brain bleed and seizure. I was unconscious for about forty-five minutes.

When I began to "come to," I didn't know where I was, who anyone was, or what had happened. Happily, I quickly remembered who people were. My husband was already at the hospital with me, but my three oldest children and extended family members were called to immediately come to the hospital. At this point, the doctors were unsure about the second brain bleed. Was I going to make it? Was I going to need surgery? The doctors didn't yet have answers. Thankfully, the bleed did stop, I didn't need surgery, and I'm alive today to tell this story.

This has been, and continues to be, *hard*. I am blessed and so very thankful to be alive, but I'm also scared, and angry, and frustrated, but I am also determined and hopeful. Sometimes I'm sad, and realistic, and impatient, and exhausted, and in constant pain, and embarrassed, and relieved, and peaceful, and unsure, and confused. *Every single day is difficult, and every single day is unpredictable.*

I am in constant pain. On a scale of 1 to 10, I stay between a 6 and a 9, every day. I'm always dizzy, off-balance, and sometimes I feel like I'm going to fall. It seems like I'm constantly trying to focus and refocus my eyes, or squinting, just trying to be able to see what I'm reading, or what's going on around me. I'm unable to drive a vehicle—and to a mother of six, that is a very frustrating problem. I have cognitive deficits, but nobody seems to understand those at all. At any given time, I struggle with short-term memory, word finding, getting "lost" mid-sentence or in thought, and I forget simple words that I used to know, that I *should* know. I'm not who I used to be. I could go on and on, and give other problems, more examples, but if you have a traumatic brain injury, you already know what I'm talking about.

So, what do we do? Why am I writing this? TBI survivors all seem to say and write similar things about our struggles. It's good to vent, to have other people like you who you can share your story and your frustrations with.

But, what do we *need*?

✱Find a way to understand.

- We need the people around us to be educated about what we're *really* going through—the daily, sometimes minute-to-minute struggles that we face, that we can't put into words, no matter how many articles we read.
- We can't tell our loved ones what we need, or how to help us, because our brains won't let us form the right group of words to get it out of our mouths.
- We don't want or need any more sympathy.
- We need the people around us to find a way to understand that we're trapped inside our own brains.
- We need you to understand that just because our bruises and cuts are healed, and we "look" okay, *we're not okay!* This is a daily struggle. And, sometimes, it's a nightmare.
- We're not lazy, we're not ignoring you...we're using every ounce of our now depleted brain-energy to just even resemble some kind of "peace and normal."

We need you to, on your own, research *legitimate* medical information and read stories of other TBI survivors, so you can *try* to help us verbalize what is going on inside of our brains, and to *try* to understand how *frustrating, frightening, and lonely* this journey is. For me, it's kind of like those old "20/20" specials. They showed a patient being put under for surgery, but the anesthesia doesn't work, so the patient can feel every cut that's being made, but he can't open his eyes or mouth to let anyone know, so he lies there, in agonizing pain. That's what this is like.

Exactly.

On those days that our pain level is so high, we're so exhausted, the brain fog and the confusion is so thick, and we just can't find our way, caregivers and family members that have the knowledge of what signs to look for and how to offer realistic "help," would make all the difference in the life of a person with traumatic brain injury. We don't need jokes, or to be told to "get over it," or that *you're* "tired of hearing about" our brain injury, or to be left alone to deal with everything...*alone*.

We already feel alone, being trapped inside our own brains, knowing and remembering how we used to be...emotionally, mentally, and physically—and knowing that *that* person is *never* coming back. Well-meaning doctors, physical therapists, and speech therapists say, "Be patient...be patient." We don't need or want our family and friends to tell us that same, sterile message. We aren't stupid; we realize that we have to be patient; *there's no other option*! We need you to realize that we are pushing ourselves, emotionally, mentally, and physically, as hard as we can, and then some, and sometimes, too far, which takes *days* to recover.

So, my message to my family and friends, and to other traumatic brain injury survivors' families and friends is simple: *All we need is just a little patience, love, and respect.*

Amy Hastings is a stay-at-home momma. She is forty-three, and has six children, ages three to seventeen. She believes that in all things, God is always and actively working for our good.

Chapter Seven
On a Dime

Amy London
Phoenix, Arizona

My name is Amy, and I am a brain injury survivor. It seems so peculiar to be writing this story, so unjustified, even to myself. You see, I am one of the individuals I've heard classified as the "walking wounded," "the invisible illness," or "the forgotten people."

You wouldn't know to look at me that anything is amiss—I can walk, talk, and communicate in complete sentences. By today's societal standards, I appear quite functional and relatively well. So well, in fact, you would never imagine the stunning amount of resources I am expending just to meet you intellectually where you are at—and that's on a good day.

Then maybe, just maybe, for the 10 minutes we converse, you might presume I'm just like my old self again and all is well, but I've come to terms with the fact there are many cracks and crevices in a 24-hour day for another, very different, Amy to appear. This Amy is moody and at times much more disconcerting and difficult to deal with. She cannot discern between the severity of losing her keys or losing her car. She painstakingly forages for words, and then falteringly forces them out as if they were passing through thick pads of cotton. She mistakes the past for the present, and then fails to recognize the future as something to look forward to, instead of feared.

So these are the very things, among many others, which still render me incapable of asserting, even simply to myself, this is going to go away—that this "brain injury thing," this "time I hit my head," is not so minute. *Just because I am still in one piece, without any obvious physical or mental damage, it doesn't mean I am completely whole.*

If only I had gone in the other room for a ladder.

In the late evening of July 2015, dinner was cooking in my kitchen oven while I was reading a book outside on my porch. As it was summertime in the southwest, the heat seemed relentless, so I was trying my best not to be inside while the oven was on. Every so often I would open the small, windowed porch door and glance in to check the timer and see how long my dinner had left to cook. It was a minor inconvenience, but I felt especially irritable. It had been a trying day, and I was still unsettled even after an evening bout of rigorous swimming.

After one particular peek I closed the door, and as I sat back down with my book I heard a very strange sound of "bzzbapt, bzzbapt, bzzbapt," coming from the kitchen. Startled, I peered in the window of the door and saw the silhouette of a cicada hitting the thickly glassed dome light in the kitchen. I groaned, knowing full well what a pain it was going be to extricate this insect from my home, since it was not only large, but also flying and full of frantic energy. Sighing loudly I placed my book in the chair, plodded inside, and started surveying the room, planning what to do next.

This is where I would like to go back in my time machine.

It took me a while to locate the crafty creature, which had decided to take a break and cease its self-injurious behavior long enough to perch quite comfortably on the upper ridge of the tall kitchen cupboards. After evaluating that squashing it would create too much of a distasteful mess, I gathered my designated "bug-to-go" plastic cup and lid so I could transport it back out into the free world. But I needed to get up there somehow in order to reach it.

No sooner did the thought enter my mind than my eyes landed on one of the high-backed barstool chairs used at my breakfast table. Exceedingly tall for a chair, it suddenly seemed like a perfect candidate for the job. I scooted it over to the cabinet with the back facing away from me, delicately holding the cup and lid in hand, and climbed on top of the seat.

You do know what happens next, don't you?

Curiously, the cicada was caught very easily. I dropped the cup over it, and carefully slid the lid underneath so as not to disturb it, but it sat very quiet and still, as if it surreptitiously knew somehow things were not going to go well from here. I was so engrossed in keeping the cup and the lid steady so it couldn't escape, that when I proceeded to step backwards off said exceedingly tall chair, I didn't take into consideration that I was up off the floor three times higher than an average chair. My body and brain didn't either.

I remember falling as if it were orchestrated...so fast I didn't equate any fear with what was happening. The first "crack" I heard was my tailbone hitting the kitchen's ceramic stone tile floor. The foot I attempted to step down with had slipped out right from under me, and my tailbone took the initial blow. The second "crack" I heard was the back of my skull hitting the brick wall in my kitchen. Picture an L-shaped landing, only one where it suddenly and awkwardly rotates 45 degrees counterclockwise.

==And just like that, everything changed.==

They say your life can turn on a dime, or suddenly change when you least expect it. That night, and in the few weeks and even months that followed, I didn't really grasp just how true that was going to be for me moving forward. After all, you have to be knocked out to have a concussion, right? You have to throw up to have a concussion, right? You have to be slurring and stumbling and bleeding profusely to have a concussion, right? And while we're at it, it is called a concussion, right? Well, then, what's with this "traumatic brain injury" stuff? You mentioned mild… is there also an option of medium and hot? Yes, I'll take mine to go with an order of nachos on the side, please.

Needless to say, I had no idea what I'd just fallen into.

The first few weeks I spent most of my time adjusting to the fact that I, the most self-sufficient, technologically savvy, independent individual in my family was now going to have to live with little-to-no access to a computer, cell phone, or car, because all things light, sound, and smell resulted in chaos, confusion, dizziness, nausea, or burning headaches so unbearable I imagined there must be little elves lighting matchsticks with unbridled glee in my frontal lobe.

Simple, ordinary, everyday tasks like writing down directions seemed dauntingly overwhelming, and information overload was an enormous understatement. If there were any secondary distractions, such as in-store background music or overhead fluorescent lighting, forget it, I felt like an infant left immobilized in the midst of a busy intersection. Full meltdown included.

So armed with a pen and paper, off I went off in search of assistance.

It fascinated and disheartened me how little information was available on mild traumatic brain injury recovery, or rather, how difficult it was for me to find it. Right then I set an intention, upon recovery, to be part of that solution, however small. Fortunately I was graced with good health insurance so I did ultimately uncover a neurologist who worked with a team of rehabilitative specialists, and alongside that, additional physicians to assist with my recovery.

But I did have to face other dealings of this suddenly new daily regime, including the mishaps and mix-ups of disability paperwork, the concerns in continuing my leave of employment, the search for safe and reliable transportation, and the juggling of going from zero to ten prescriptions a day, in what seemed like overnight.

And quite often, in the still moments, I felt exhausted, in pain, lonely, and afraid. *all the time...*

For a single person on her own without anyone to help consistently, it was regularly a struggle to sustain momentum, and to keep fortitude and faith that everything would work out and be okay. Many evenings when I gently held my head before falling sleep, I wasn't sure I was willing to wake up, as if by choice I could determine the outcome one way or another. This is not to say I didn't have any moral support, but I felt no one around me could specifically relate to the emotions I was feeling, or the physical symptoms I was experiencing. The doctors alluded to timeframes for healing, yet in their offices I had trouble understanding everything they told me.

Was that three months?

Am I supposed to take this for four or eight days?

What about these zinging electrical surges playing tag under my scalp?

Do you…? Are you…? Can you…?

Ad infinitum.

I have no idea how I did it initially when I was so dazed and confused, only to say that I'm certain I didn't, not on my own. I can't quite place it without sounding philosophical or waxing poetic, but even in the thickest, darkest moments there seemed to be something at my core preventing me from giving up entirely:

- Even 7 weeks later, when after a rear-end car accident I began experiencing aphasia-like episodes along with a stutter;
- Even 5 weeks after that, when following a chiropractic cervical adjustment, painful paresthesia, (numbness and tingling), in my legs and feet prohibited me from walking from one end of the grocery store to another;
- Even 9 weeks after that, when I experienced prescription side effects so severe I needed medical intervention; and
- Even 6 weeks after that, when in the wake of an emotional collapse, I was forced to reexamine my definition of the word "recovery."

Now this is the part where, despite all the trials and tribulations, everything eventually works out, doesn't it? Well…yes, sort of.

My journey is far from over. In fact, in the brain injury world where time in and of itself seems to function by very strange scientific laws, they say it's just beginning. Healing here isn't always linear, it can be random and appear in doubtful or distinctive spurts. Although this process has, at times, felt long and painfully arduous, and even been met with challenges and setbacks, I've also been graced with gifts that are ever so slowly being revealed. It really all depends on how you look at it.

It's true, I am a different Amy, more of a mosaic than a solid block of stone, and I recognize now that things will never be "better," they will merely be "different." How I interpret the rest is up to me. Of course I didn't want to write this story from personal experience, but here I am, and there you are, and together we share the commonality of coincidence, however small or uncertain.

Together perhaps this story can help us understand each other just a little bit better, and brain injury a little bit more. Together each time I speak up and acknowledge my brain injury, and you recognize that it comes in all shapes and sizes, we raise awareness and inspire others to do the same. Together when you are beside me, I feel supported, and we remind each other we are not alone. Together at the very least, we can always remember… go get a ladder.

Amy London is an Arizona native and an adoptive caretaker to an outdoor cat who curiously appeared in the weeks immediately following her brain injury. Formerly active in web design, theatre, film and music, Amy has gratefully found a different kind of footing in the arts through painting, drawing, and creative writing. She can be found online at www.amylondon.com.

Chapter Eight
Noggin Nonsense:
The Harder the Hit...

Amy Pilotte
Manchester, New Hampshire

On July 12, 2014, I was the happiest and healthiest *I've ever been*. I didn't take any supplements, ate healthy foods, worked out five or six days a week, and was physically active. I could multitask, drive across country solo, and do just about anything I put my mind to.

After I decided to put myself first at the end of a long, toxic and unhealthy relationship, I began to love life and everything in it—*including myself!* I started to follow what made me happy, pushed fear aside, and jumped head first into my passions. I decided to leave my lifelong career in the corporate world and start my career as an esthetician. I had to build both a clientele and my confidence while making a complete career change—which was extremely hard and a huge growing process for me. All during this time I juggled two bartending jobs, which meant I was on the go nonstop, up at 5 a.m., at the gym every day, and off to multiple jobs every week. I rarely took time off, and was 100 percent focused on myself and on rebuilding my future.

Not even three miles from my house, I was at a dead stop in my car, waiting to merge, when I was rear-ended. Thankfully I was wearing my seatbelt; however, from what I recall I did hit my head on the steering wheel. Due to looking left at the time of impact in order to merge, I also received two herniated discs in my neck.

I had taken July 12th off to celebrate a co-worker's birthday. This would be my first time ever with them outside of work in two years. Both my best friend was visiting from California, and my cousin from

Chicago, so it was a jam-packed week. I got ready to go out, hopped in my car and was on my way.

I remember it clear as day. Needless to say, I never made it out that night.

You know that quote, "Life happens while you're making other plans?" Well, it couldn't be any more than the truth.

First I was told I received a "concussion," which later turned into a TBI, along with Post-Concussive Syndrome and two herniated discs in my neck. I'm beyond thankful and blessed it wasn't worse, no matter how hard some days can be. My life as I knew it, and had worked so hard for, was completely flipped upside down in the matter of seconds. Some days it still doesn't seem real. I just make the best of it and roll with the punches.

Since my accident two years ago, my relationship with every single person in my life has changed. Many people don't know *what a TBI means for me*. They feel like I can just "snap out of it." Many doctors don't have experience with TBIs, and don't understand that every case is different and based on the individual. Lack of services from the community is also frustrating, and without a caseworker, it is very difficult to fill out forms, make appointments, keep track of medications, and figure out rides. This all makes for a lot of unnecessary stress, and it takes away from other activities that I could be working on to help with my recovery. I think many people feel that since they can't "see" my disability, it can't be that bad. However, to this day, it takes everything I have *to get out of bed each morning*.

Recovery has been the worst rollercoaster of my life, but I'm hanging on and riding along. No one tells you that recovery is *long*, and that's the worst part of all. Presently, at the two-year mark, my speech is better. After seeing so many different doctors that I had lost count, I finally have a team of medical professionals that have me on the right track with medication, procedures, and rehabilitation. I listen to my body more now; it knows best. When I need rest, I need rest. I have to be honest with my support system—and myself—about how I feel from day to day. Putting me first is a daily priority and necessity.

Life has changed in every way possible. It's hard to have to depend on people for so much when I've always been very independent and self-sufficient. I'm still unable to drive or work. My executive and cognitive functions were affected, and there is no way to tell when and if they will return to 100 percent. I feel drastically different from when I first had my accident, and even though I'm nowhere near the same, I'm very thankful for the progress I've made. There have been many hurdles, and there will be many more, but I have the determination to keep going. Every little step counts in my recovery, and I'm forever thankful for the little things these days. I'm especially grateful to the people who have supported and stood by my side every single step of the way.

Happy New Life Day! Wowee! That first year was a blur, the second year has been a struggle, but I know deep down *The Best is yet to come*, Cheers to staying Strong and Keeping on!

Amy Pilotte is a brain injury survivor living in New England with her family while continuing to focus on recovering. During her recovery and new walk of life, she plans to continue to raise as much awareness as possible, and remain an active member of the TBI Tribe.

Chapter nine
Finding the Right Treatment and Doctors Has Been a 19-Year Struggle

Anne Forrest
Austin, Texas

My new sports doctor said, "Our goal is to get you to zero symptoms."

After 19 years of searching for appropriate care following a mild traumatic brain injury (mTBI) caused by a car accident near Lincoln Memorial in Washington, DC in 1997, I was finally hearing the words that I had never even known to ask for. With poor cognitive skills from the injury, this was music to my ears. Oh…there is my goal, and I am almost there. Once I had sufficient awareness to understand that without any cognitive rehab treatment to help me resolve my concussion symptoms, I had to use whatever skills I had to continue to live my life.

Now I had to find *a new me*, under the worst of circumstances. My brain that was so important to me, no longer worked right, and getting through the day took tremendous effort and forbearance. So many days I was ready to throw in the towel. Recovering from brain injury was like trying to live one's life, just with tremendous barriers, like brain malfunctions that I didn't understand, and many others around me, including some of my colleagues, couldn't see at first.

I looked fine to many of them, but I couldn't drive, and I was too fatigued to do more than one thing in a day. I also needed help eating, and with my own safety

In my apartment one day, I remember thinking that if this could happen to me…what was it like for others who didn't have my advantages. I grew up middle class, and had the advantages of a great education at Yale, and Duke where I obtained a PhD. At the time of my accident, I had car insurance, work disability insurance that I had never looked at, and health insurance. Trying to find care with my injury was a Catch-22. If I didn't have the injury, I could have explained why I needed care and what kind of care. But now my brain didn't know enough to identify—and what to ask.

That day in the apartment, I recall thinking that I had to get well to help others, because if *this was as good as it gets,* what was it like for others? My advocacy was born that afternoon.

I had a lot of other help from colleagues who got it, or sort of got it. We set up a system to make sure I didn't fall into a "dark pit," and were never seen again, since I lived alone. I saw some of the best doctors I could find. When I realized I couldn't read, my network found me an optometrist who did vision therapy and began the process of re-teaching me. He said my brain could heal, despite my neurologist and primary care doctor's warnings that *what I didn't get back in two years, I would never get back.* They had also expected me to be back to work in 3–6 months. I was a PhD economist who now couldn't add up my time sheet. The chief finance officer knew, and asked me to go out on disability.

My friend's dad got me in to see a doctor in New York City who understood that neurooptometric vision therapy issues came with traumatic brain injury. He recommended doctors and specialists in Washington, D.C., but when I saw those doctors, they did not seem to understand my needs the way the New York City doctor thought—so I received some help, but not all I needed.

Finally, 3½ years later, St. David's Rehabilitation Hospital in Austin, Texas, accepted me for outpatient cognitive rehabilitation. It, along with the continued vision therapy, turned my life around.

When I first had my injury, my friends, family and many colleagues, as well as several doctors, did not know one could have prolonged symptoms after a mild traumatic brain injury/concussion. Like me, they did not know that the "mild" diagnosis could still be severe and long lasting. I had to find the best doctors who believed that if I were not able to live my life or do my job, appropriate treatment would help—and I did respond to appropriate treatment, when I could get it.

I found that my health insurance would pay for the right treatments, just often not enough. Despite my health insurance paying for it, other insurance companies (work disability and car insurance) questioned whether *I had just decided to live off the dole*, and thus sent me to doctors who supported their point of view. I had to look up words they ascribed to me, like "histrionic" and "malingerer." These companies had accepted my money or my employer's money for insurance premiums when I was well, but now when it was their time to pay out for the policy, they found reasons not to help. It was an incredible distraction from getting well and getting back to work, which is what I wanted.

St. David's Rehabilitation Hospital accepted me for rehab. I asked a social worker there why they were treating me, if in fact, my brain couldn't get better after 2 years. With the vision therapy and chiropractic care, I was getting better, just not enough, and I knew it, but I wanted to understand why I had been told my brain couldn't get better. The social worker said he thought *people just give up because the system is just too oppressive*.

Once I got to cognitive rehabilitation my therapists told me they believed in neuroplasticity—that my brain could rewire, and I could get better. After a year of therapy, my insurance would no longer pay. I became a volunteer with Dr. John Slatin at the University of Texas; then called the Institute for Technology and Learning, now is known as Office of Accessibility. I gave my first speech—the speech I had written with my cognitive therapist. It was to help develop my awareness of my injury, and to develop my language skills to protect myself from people that thought I was fine. I gave this speech to Dr. Slatin's class in 2001. Speaking was my transferable skill, according to my cognitive therapist who assessed my current abilities side-by-side with me. I also taught a class called, "Accessibility of the Internet for People with Cognitive Disabilities"—I was the case study of TBI. Pre-injury, I had spoken about sustainable development to people around the world, now I was learning about my own sustainable development through speaking. Dr. Slatin, who had become blind in graduate school, launched my speaking career.

My husband and I were married in Austin in 2001. He had been my biggest supporter after my injury. In 2002, we returned to Washington, D.C. traumatic brain injury had become the signature injury—and awareness grew due to injuries incurred during the Gulf War (1990–1991). Later, Congress forced the NFL to alert players about potential damage to their head from playing football.

My cousin told me to listen to Trisha Meilli, who wrote "I Am the Central Park Jogger: A Story of Hope and Possibility," speak about her book on the Diane Rehm show on National Public Radio (NPR). Moments after hearing the show, the "Washington Post" called to ask if I would tell my story for their column, "Coping with Challenges." Through going to see Trisha Meilli at a bookstore, I was connected with the Brain Injury Association of America (BIAA) through a social worker. When I visited BIAA, a person with brain injury who volunteered there suggested I use the second desk in his office.

I had my first start back to work; I had a desk. My skill level was challenged by just getting to BIAA by bus once a week. I had more rehab at Inova Mt. Vernon Rehabilitation Hospital. I spoke with Brain Injury Services of Northern Virginia Speakers Bureau. "The Washingtonian Magazine" wrote an article about living with Brain Injury that has helped people from around the world, and is still a major resource on living with brain injury. The article, "I Wanted My Brain Back: What happens when you're a PhD economist and you suddenly can't remember things of think straight? One woman's story of perseverance reveals some of the mysteries of the brain."
BIAA gave me the opportunity to speak at their State-of-the-Art Post-Acute Rehabilitation conference as an opener for Claudia Osborn, D.O. Claudia had been my idol for rehab after I found her book two years after my injury. She wrote, "Over My Head: A Doctor's Own Story of Head Injury from the Inside Looking Out." Then-BIAA President Alan Bergmann told me they were looking for a survivor who had not received any rehab for two years following the injury, and who had gotten better. That was my story! I became an evangelist for neuroplasticity. Attendees Drs. Robin Green and

Margaret Weiser asked me to come to Toronto, Canada to speak.

I have now given over 60 speeches where I talk about my ongoing recovery, the difficulties of getting care for people with concussion and cognitive accessibility. I was one of the first regular civilian (not sports or military-related) to speak on the Congressional Brain Injury Panel on Capitol Hill for Brain Injury Awareness day in 2011, and received a standing ovation. In 2016, I was on a panel at the One Mind Summit with several MDs and PhDs about "The Case for Standardized Screening for Concussion in the Emergency Departments in the US."

Now after 19 years, my doctor is telling me that I will be "well," with more rehab, and *it is music to my ears*! A week later, I received the newsletter from Memorial Hermann Hospital in Houston saying,
> "Fifteen years ago, the approach to treating concussion was almost laissez-faire: a few days of bed rest, then back to normal activity. Our knowledge of concussion has increased exponentially in the last 10 years… there is a new awareness that structured, individualized, progressive aerobic exercise may reduce symptoms of post concussive symptoms… early intervention reduces symptoms and accelerates the course of recovery, but patients at any stage of recovery benefit from a structured multidisciplinary plan of care." – TIRR Memorial Hermann Journal Newsletter, Summer 2016.

And my path to recovery has benefitted from the wisdom and insight of other supporters, in addition to Trisha Meilli and Claudia Osborne who I have already mentioned. In 2008, Susan Connors, President and CEO, of BIAA gathered together 5 people with brain injuries to form a group that would advise BIAA. I was one of them. We worked with Susan for three or four phone calls, then set out on our own to charter a group. At the time, we encountered major problems with organization, simply remembering what was said in the last call, causing some to drop off the call. We realized that because we had the injury, organization would be tough, but it was an opportunity we couldn't let go. Today, we have eight active, dedicated members on the group as well as our liaison to BIAA. We have helped revitalize patient participation at BIAA, helped with the redesign of BIAA website into more accessible information chunks, and are launching a nationwide speaker's bureau so that people looking for speakers can find those with life experience. As chair of this group, I have been blessed to work with and benefit tremendous wisdom and inspiration from our group, and know that we are inspiring others.

And a year ago, I benefitted from being asked to help with the Diane Rehm NPR program on "New Therapies for Concussion," working with Clark Elliott, a PhD with a concussion who recovered after 8 years. Elliott wrote, "The Ghost in My Brain: How the New Science of Brain Plasticity Helped Me Get It Back."

Listening to the final program, I realized I was doing all the right things Clark Elliot did—cognitive rehab and neurooptometry. When he found these treatments, he had a 70 percent recovery in two months after having had no treatment for 8 years after his injury. I was doing the right things—I just had to do more of them! What motivation. If he could do it, so could I.

I have received vestibular and then neurooptometric therapy, this time at St. David's Outpatient Rehabilitation Hospital, and have made tremendous progress. I feel like my brain is an inch bigger, I am able to organize in ways I haven't been able to, and am much more functional. It hasn't been easy, but it can be done. *I am getting there after 19 years.* After switching doctors, my new doctor is telling me that the end of the tunnel is in sight! Really.

An accessibility expert is helping me so that the computer is not a barrier to me, and in exchange for his help, he wants to learn from me about concussion, neurooptometric rehab, and Neuroplasticity.

My blog, www.APlasticBrain.com is accessible to others like me who have neurooptometric issues after a concussion.

Anne Forrest, PhD, is the Chair of the Brain Injury Advisory Council (BIAC), a collaborative effort between leaders with brain injuries and the Brain Injury Association of America. She speaks about her recovery and blogs on her website www.aplasticbrain.com

Chapter Ten
The Best Thing About Miracles Is That They Happen

Austin Clayton Craft
Knightstown, Indiana

In June of 2014, I graduated from Knightstown High School. Most of my free time I worked out at the Anytime Fitness gym in Greenfield, Indiana. I was just starting to prepare to compete in my first bodybuilding show that November.

On December 2, 2014, I left the gym to go to my dad's house. It was dark and foggy, and I pulled out in front of a semi-truck going about 55 mph. My pickup truck was crushed, and it took them over an hour to get me out of the truck. They took me to Methodist Hospital and induced me into a coma. I had a diffuse axonal brain injury, and also suffered a shearing brain injury. On the third day of being there, I coded and my heart stopped beating. They gave me an adrenaline shot, and my heart started to beat again.

The doctors said I would be in vegetative state, and three different times asked my family if they wanted to terminate the care for me. Luckily they didn't give up—and this is what motivates me more than anything. After about a month, I woke up from my coma, and after two months, I was released to go home from the hospital. After being home for one week, I returned to the Anytime Fitness gym. I have slowly worked my way back up, and I am now stronger and bigger than I was before my accident. The day I went home from the hospital, I was 157 pounds and today I am around 215 pounds.

It was very hard to work my way back up because I was very little and weak—and I also had double vision, making it even harder. I was always scared that I would go too hard and end up hurting myself. So for the whole first year, I took it easy. I pushed myself a little harder throughout the year. But I didn't go all out until one year after my accident. Fitness has been huge for me and has been a big part of my recovery. I would say for me that working out and staying in shape is why I am recovering so well. Honestly they told my family at the hospital that was a reason I survived the wreck.

I hope to achieve my dream and compete in my first bodybuilding show in spring of 2018.

I have started college again after a year of being out of school. I am majoring in kinesiology at Ivy Tech. My goal is to one day become a personal trainer. My first semester I took two classes, Psychology and English and I got an A and a B. I worked really hard, and I am proud.

I have tried to motivate and inspire others since my accident. I have shown my progress photos in the group TBI Tribe on Facebook. My grandma suffered a stroke and is going through therapy and rehabilitation, and I have tried to inspire her to do her best and show her that it is possible to recover. Also, my friend on my basketball team in high school was in a car crash, and he is now recovering after being in the hospital for two months. It obviously has been really hard for his family, and they tell me that I give them hope. That means a lot!

It's really been hard for me and other TBI survivors—but the best thing in the world is knowing that *you are a survivor*!

Austin is 20 years old and lives in Knightstown, Indiana. He continues to train at Anytime Fitness and plans to compete in his first body building competition in the spring of 2018.

Chapter Eleven
Brought to My Knees

Barbara Myers
Laguna Niguel, California

September 28, 2015…It was a day like any other day for this incredibly busy woman. I remember that I was running late for an appointment as I hurried out of my office and decided to stop by the bathroom before heading to my appointment. I was wearing a dress, something I don't often do, and flat sandals. I had my bag slung over my shoulder but nothing in my hands. As I walked briskly up the four stone steps to the bathroom, I missed a step and went flying. Picture Superman as that is what I looked like. I tried to get my hands down but couldn't do it fast enough, and bam! I landed at the top of the stairs, specifically where the stone step met the industrial carpet, only I landed on my chin. I remember my head snapping back violently. Nothing else on my body bore the brunt of my fall. The underside of my chin absorbed the entire impact.

All I remember next is some bald man sprinting out of the office that is next to the bathroom. In an instant, he was trying to help me as I stood up. "Are you okay?" he asked. "Yeah, I'm fine. That's what I get for rushing," I replied with an embarrassed laugh. I made it to the restroom, briefly cried while in the stall, wiped my eyes and went to my appointment. I came back to work, kept on working, but at 5:00 I turned to my husband whom I worked with, and cried. My chin really hurt. My neck was killing me. I cried for a few minutes, wiped my eyes and kept working. Fast forward to the next day. I drove into work with a splitting headache. I lasted for less than five minutes before the world started spinning, and I thought I would be sick. That afternoon I was diagnosed with my second concussion and severe whiplash. At the time of my diagnosis, I wasn't too concerned.

My first concussion happened over 20 years ago. I was playing tennis with my husband, doubles to be exact, when he went for an overhead, didn't see me, and whacked me hard on top of the head with his racquet. Please understand that this was no small thing being that my husband and I had been playing tennis since we were small children. He played in college and hit hard. Very hard. It took me about a month but I fully but I fully recovered. I had no idea of what awaited me with this second concussion. I didn't understand how serious concussions could be. I left work on September 28, 2015, and I didn't return to work until January 2016. This injury brought this wellness coach and escrow officer to her knees, and I am only just now starting to stand again.

What followed was months of headaches, dizziness, sensitivity to any kind of light or loud noise, neuro-fatigue, and an inability to follow conversations or complex problems. I went from exercising six days a week to barely being able to get out of bed. I couldn't do anything. No reading. No computer time. No cooking. I was exhausted and so dizzy. I was allowed to watch TV, but nothing requiring thought. I don't watch a lot of stupid TV. I love documentaries, but watching a documentary was out of the question. I remember telling the doctor I was going to watch "Breaking Bad," and was told I couldn't because it was too cerebral. I was reduced to watching Army Wives... Army Wives. Seriously? I remember watching a lot of sports. Thank God for football season.

I remember telling my husband that he had to slow down when speaking to me. I told him this all the time, and I still have to from time to time even now. I am also always telling him to turn down the TV, radio, whatever, because the noise bothers me. To this day, I still can't go the grocery store. All the boxes and colors and rows and rows of products make me dizzy. I wear sunglasses at night after a long day at work. I feel like a gangster as I roll down the freeway in my car.

I mean, come on! How ridiculous is this? I just fell, for heaven's sake! This goes through my mind constantly. The worst symptom for me was the inability to think as quickly. I am known for my quick thinking. I deal with hundreds, literally hundreds, of emails every day, but once I fell, I couldn't do a damn thing. I close and balance files all day long. I multitask constantly. I do math and figure out problems for a living, and after I fell, I could barely think. It was awful, and I felt like a complete waste of space. I remember wondering if I would ever feel normal again. If I am honest, I still worry about this today.

One of the symptoms that I was not warned about was the complete inability to sleep. Every night I would lie awake, exhausted but unable to sleep. At the beginning, I slept all day and night, but as time went on, I couldn't sleep at all. My Fitbit would register my sleep patterns, and I would check it out each morning. Awake 13 times and restless 58 times per night became the norm. It was awful. I couldn't stay asleep to save my soul. It's October now and finally my sleep is returning to a more normal pattern. I have good days and bad days but the good days are starting to outnumber the bad days. Progress.

Eventually I had to go back to work, so back I went in January. Besides dealing with the fact that I was struggling to be able to even perform my job, I had to deal with coworkers not understanding what was happening to me. "You look great! You're better now, right?" "Everything is fine now, right?" "Why can't you be in on the conference call after your four hours or work? It's just a conference call?"

In all fairness, they just didn't understand my injury. Very few people do. I had restricted work hours but I did not have enough help to enable me to keep to the restrictions. I basically worked full time the entire time, no matter how dizzy I was. This part of the recovery was the absolute worst for me. I looked fine. I made an effort every day to put on my makeup, get dressed, smile and not complain, so I must have been fine, right? I dreaded people asking me how I was feeling because I could see the looks on their faces when I told them I still wasn't fine. I could see how puzzled they were. I looked fine. I laughed. I was working. How could I still be injured? They just didn't get it. Some looked like they didn't believe me. Some never even asked me how I was. I felt misunderstood, doubted and very hurt. A few cared enough to try and understand what had happened to me. My eyes welled with tears every time one of those few actually stopped by my office to talk to me and encourage me. As I type this, my eyes are filling with tears. Those people were like angels to me. and I will never forget their kindness and support.

I was so stressed out about work that I ended up with a full-blown anxiety disorder. Every day as I hit the freeway to go to work, my pulse would start to race. During the work day, my chest would literally hurt from how hard my heart was pounding. There were times I started to cry at my desk because I was so overwhelmed by what I had to do. I found out later that this was called flooding and I still deal with this regularly. Flooding is when everything hits you all at once because your brain can't filter stimuli as well. It's a very scary feeling. I had to go on medication to stabilize my heart rate and blood pressure. I wasn't prepared for that as I am active and fit, and those issues have never been a part of my life. Once again, I felt like a failure. My life became all about surviving the workweek. No exercise. No cooking dinner. Nothing. I just got through the workweek, and on the weekends, I slept. I slept like the dead. I did nothing fun, and didn't go anywhere. Nothing. I had to completely shut down to get ready for the next week. My husband of twenty-five years was the best. He never complained. He sat with me and rubbed my feet. He went out to get dinner. He worked harder than ever to try and lessen my load. He let me rage with frustration, and held me when I sobbed, thinking I would never have my life back. He is the single reason I came through this and his support is unwavering even now. Our weekends are still spent helping me recover. He still never complains and is right beside me every step of the way.

That was my injury, but I did not let it define me. I am so much more than my injury. I joined Run the Year 2016, which is a challenge to walk 2016 miles in 2016. I already know that won't make it, but it gave me something to shoot for with my exercise. I have stopped and started exercise routines more times than I can remember this year, but I never quit and I never will. I logged all my food in LoseIt. I made sure to make good choices with what I ate, and I have not gained weight. I kept at it until I was able to be active again. After a year spent trying to find an exercise that I can do, I finally discovered stationary biking. I can cycle because my head doesn't bounce around. I am also able to practice gentle yoga now. Finding an exercise program that I can do helped me deal with my stress and anxiety which is big progress. As for work, I am much better. I still deal with daily dizziness and flooding but I am able to cope better. The headaches don't happen all the time now, but when they do, they seem to come in clusters. I will have a headache all day every single day for days. Most recently I went through a six day period of this. Nothing helps but sleep and I can't sleep during the workday. I have learned to live with them. I choose to focus on how far I've come, not how far I have to go.

I was discharged from the doctor the other day. I am not fully recovered, but the rest of my recovery is up to me. I need to make sure I get enough rest. I need to listen to my body, and stop when it tells me to stop. The medical profession can't help me with that. I have always pushed past physical limitations, but I can't push past this. Finding the time to rest and taking the time that I need to heal has been and continues to be the greatest challenge for me. I struggle with this but I am getting better at it. Perhaps that is the blessing in all of this. My injury helped me *to learn that it is okay to rest.*

I hope that anyone who reads this is inspired—inspired to never quit, and inspired to keep fighting no matter how bleak it seems. I know I am one of the lucky ones. I know my injury could have been so much worse. I could have broken my neck and died. I am here. I am healthy. I am a work in progress. I will never quit and I will recover 100 percent! Nothing will stop me; don't let anything or anyone stop you.

Barb is a 52-year-old wife, mother, health and wellness coach, and escrow officer. Her job is demanding and pressure filled, but she continues to find ways to cope with her symptoms. She is determined to fully recover and to enjoy all life has to offer in spite of her injury. Her motto is: Never ever quit!

Chapter Twelve
How Women Respond and React Differently to Injuries: Specifically Brain Injuries

Beth Westie, Doctor of Chiropractic
Minneapolis, MN

Overall, when we look at recovery from an injury, these few things are really important to understand:

Nutrition–Yes, nutrition plays a huge role in how fast and how well you recover from any type of injury—whether it be a traumatic brain injury or not.

Hormones–The difference that hormones play in recovery overall when it comes to gender differences is this. Men have the same hormone everyday: testosterone. Every day a man has a pretty similar amount of hormone. For women, it's very different. The levels of estrogen and progesterone change slightly day to day, but especially week to week.

Since estrogen and progesterone play such important roles in the body, this is an important piece to how this fits into recovery. Women overall are usually seen to take longer to recover from injuries, which is due to the day-to-day change in hormones.

Your body needs certain nutrients to metabolize and eliminate the excess hormone from the body. If you are not getting nutrient-dense food that is in alignment with your hormones, your organs are going to suffer. They will be unable to function at their optimal level in order to flush out and eliminate excess toxins in the body that come along with healing naturally.

When you are recovering from an injury, a certain process has to occur. When there is damage done, cells need to be repaired—and it takes energy, or nutrient to make that happen. The more nutrient-dense foods you are making, the more perfect the cell will repair. So, if there's no nutrient, when the cell tries to heal itself, it will make a damaged cell. It will not do it as quickly or perfectly as it could. Flooding your body with great nutrient that is in alignment with dominant hormones helps the body absorb the nutrient-dense food, therefore creating healthy cells.

Blood sugar levels–Your levels are also very important in terms of recovery and healing. When your blood sugar levels go up and down, you are releasing excess cortisol into your system, and this will negatively affect your healing rate. When your blood sugar gets too high, your organs have to release a bunch of insulin to help combat. If your blood sugar drops too low, your organs have to release glucagon to help combat that. It is hard on the body, especially for women, to go on a rollercoaster all day long, especially when you are trying to heal, for this can distract your body from actually focusing on healing. For women, focusing on a high-protein diet is very important. Eating healthy fats in the morning can help regulate blood sugars and support your nervous system, and eating every 2–3 hours will keep blood sugars level throughout the day.

Stress levels–With stress and cortisol level, if there are constant spikes and dips, it can be really hard on your body when you are recovering. This can decrease insulin sensitivity. Your body has a hard time absorbing the nutrients it needs to heal at the most optimal rate. Your cells are then not able to have the nutrition they need to replicate and heal.

Yes, stress also can decrease your immune function, making you more susceptible to illness. If you happen to get sick while you are trying to recover from an injury, it overloads your body and will prolong healing time. Excess levels of stress will also convert any protein you are taking in, to sugar through a process called gluconeogenesis. That also causes you to store more energy in your fat cells, contributing to on-going problems.

Alcohol intake–Alcohol can also place more stress on your body. It causes excess work for your liver, and depletes your body of the ability to absorb nutrients. It makes it harder, and slows down recovery time.

Medications–Another big issue a lot of women do not take into consideration is medications. Medications can affect hormone levels, especially medications like birth control. Opioid pain medications also alter hormone levels. When your hormones are fluctuating, you are altering your healing process.

Hormones play a huge role in tissue growth. They can play a role in different processes in the body that are vital to healing, such as hunger and sleep. It is very important to have the right nutrient to allow cells to properly recover. Just as important is getting enough sleep. If you are not getting the right kind of restful sleep, healing cannot happen to its fullest extent, and your cells will not repair themselves as perfectly.

Hormones also affect muscle repair, bone growth, and metabolism. Metabolism is important because it determines the rate at which you will be able to flush out excess toxins from your body. Inflammation can trigger other disease reactions when an injury occurs. Using nutrition that is in alignment with your hormones is vital to increasing your metabolism and decreasing inflammation after an injury.

If you've ever worked out really hard, you can relate to this kind of recovery. If you have proper hormonal messaging going on in your body, you are able to recover much quicker. You can absorb the nutrients your body needs to help rebuild muscle tissue. Your oxygen levels are high, allowing cells to get the oxygen they need to repair. You might have noticed a time when you were sick or stressed, and you tried to do a similar workout, and found your recovery time to be a lot slower. This is due to the excess hormone in the body.

Brain Injury Specifics:

Specific differences exist between men and women when it comes to a brain injury. Research has shown that the difference noticed in brain injuries between men and women starts at puberty, and ends at menopause. Women that experience a concussion or brain injury actually have a much different rate of recovery during those years. Injuries that take place before or after those time frames respond more similarly to men. This tells us that hormones play a huge role in recovery of an injury, and especially in brain injuries.

The difference is explained by estrogen. Estrogen exacerbates the injury in women, while in men it protects the brain from the injury. However, progesterone appears to be neuroprotective. This links to the entire female cycle, and it determines how women will recover from a brain injury. Another interesting fact is that research has shown the rate of concussions in women is much higher than that of men. This again could be due to excess levels of estrogen in women.

In terms of symptoms of brain injuries, during certain phases of the female cycle, recovery can tend to take longer. Again this is due to the excess hormone in women's bodies during certain weeks of their cycle. This is also linked to the fact that women's hormones are changing and shifting throughout the month. This inhibits their ability to recover at the same rate as their male counterpart.

Another important aspect to discuss when talking about symptoms is headaches. Almost ninety percent of people suffering from a brain injury will experience a headache. This comes into play for women when their hormones shift, and there is a drop in estrogen after ovulation. Most women experience headaches during this time; however, women with a brain injury are then more likely to experience migraines.

Early diagnosis and more aggressive treatment are necessary due to the extended recovery period for women.

Dr. Beth Westie is a chiropractor, women's health expert, and author of "Stop Your Day." She has helped thousands of women get healthier using the right nutrition to match their hormones. www.drbethwestie.com

Chapter Thirteen
Blessed by a Brain Tumor

**Brenda L. Kleinsasser
Bismarck, North Dakota**

My brain tumor journey began on September 8, 2008, when I was 48. Then a craniotomy was performed in order to remove a right frontal lobe meningioma. It was found to be non-malignant, and the surgeons were able to get it all, including the tail, which is a striking characteristic of this type of brain tumor.

I need to back up here and share a bit of background to this whole adventure. I had experienced a head injury several years prior when I had leaned too far into the refrigerator and bumped my head pretty hard. I did not get knocked out, so I never had it checked out. That was not a wise move on my part, but more on that later.

My head pain got better as the months progressed, so I figured that maybe it was bruised, but life went on. The next year however, just after my father had passed away from Alzheimer's disease, the head pain started to get worse again, so I was sent to a neurologist to see what might be going on. All he did was send me home with exercises, as he was pretty sure that it was trauma from the prior head injury, and needed time to heal. He did say that a CAT scan or CT could be performed, but nothing was likely to be found. Little did we know—that was not the case.

I went home and did the exercises, and again, it did seem to get better. However, over the course of the next year, things began to get worse again. I asked my primary care physician at the time if I could possibly have a CT, as I was sure something was wrong. His nurse told me twice, over the phone, "If we find nothing, we are done." I decided to go ahead with the CT. A mass or lesion was found on the right frontal lobe. At this point, what we were actually dealing with was inclusive. The next step would be an MRI scheduled for that same week. Now, that same physician who was going to stop treating me actually knew something was going on. *I was not crazy!*

When I went for the MRI, I was asked if I was claustrophobic. I really was not sure, but after six minutes, I squeezed the panic button and had to get out of there. It had to be rescheduled for another day, under anesthesia. I did all right, but I got sick after from the anesthesia. So I did not get to go home right away, as they wanted to make sure I was feeling better, and I ended up resting there for several hours.

I was found to have a meningioma/brain tumor the size of a walnut. The next step would be to see a neurologist and then a neurosurgeon, if it was deemed necessary.

The next week my mother accompanied me to finally see the neurologist, and in all seriousness, it did not look good. He said it had nothing to do with that previous head injury. It had probably been there for at least twenty years, as this type of brain tumor is slow growing. Finally, he asked if I would like to see a neurosurgeon *today?* I said yes! Things were finally progressing. We walked over to the neurosurgeon's office. His assistant said he would be in shortly. He came and introduced himself, and shook our hands. That was pretty much how our encounters were throughout this whole process. He sat down with me and showed me the results of the MRI in-depth, non-contrast and contrast. It now looked like a comet with a tail. Nothing would be conclusive until he could look under a microscope, after the removal of the meningioma.

Surgery was scheduled for September 8, only four days away. The next day I would receive the news of how it would actually be removed. I was so clueless about so many things, but that would change quickly. When I called to pre-register for the procedure, and the nurse mentioned the word craniotomy, I said, "You mean my head is going to be drilled open." She asked, "How did you expect that it would be removed?" WOW! This *was not what I expected to hear.* I would certainly learn so much more as time went on.

I arrived at the hospital on September 8, 2008 at 6:00 a.m. It was a Monday and raining, so I sat on a bench while my mother went to park the car. This was really going to be happening.

The anesthesiologist came in and was quite frank about what could happen. He said I could experience a seizure, stroke, or could even die. He did say that they would be putting me on anti-seizure medication, to help prevent one from happening.

On the way to the operating room, my mother leaned down and kissed me on the cheek. She had never done anything like this before, so I knew she was concerned. I was now wheeled into the operating room—and my life would be forever changed.

It was to be a two-hour procedure, but it only took ninety minutes. They were able to get to the tumor quite readily, as they only had to open the bone flap. It was now the size of a golf ball, which they removed all in one piece, along with the tail. It was definitely a meningioma.

The brain tumor was located in the right frontal lobe, which made me an instant member of "a club." The right frontal lobe is considered the high-functioning level of the brain. Frontal lobe syndrome is a real thing. For the first year of my brain tumor journey, it was scary at times because I had no idea these things were normal.

I would become angry or would cry more easily, and for no reason. I finally connected with some other individuals who had gone through the same thing, and they assured me that it was perfectly normal.

One the greatest things I experienced throughout this whole journey is that I suddenly became creative. I sat down one day and wrote my first blog post. It resonated with those I shared it with, so I decided I would continue.

My mother, who was my caregiver, passed away on May 31, 2011, from congestive heart failure. My promise to her was *to live my life*. Hers was to remain in my heart. Every day, I strive to keep that promise, and sharing my story with others is a big part of that.

I am an eight-year survivor of a right frontal lobe meningioma brain tumor. Every year, when I celebrate the anniversary of my craniotomy, or "Craniversary," as what it is referred to in the brain tumor community, I know beyond a shadow of a doubt that this was all meant to happen.

My story may not be typical, but my hope is that you realize you truly can live a life after having a brain tumor. I am living proof.

Brenda L. Kleinsasser resides in Bismarck, the capital city of North Dakota. Brenda is a fierce patient advocate for both brain tumors and rheumatoid arthritis (RA), which she has lived with for over twenty-five years. Brenda enjoys writing her blog: Brenda's Brainstorm & Trevor. Trevor is her storyteller and shares tales, from a golden retriever's point of view.
www.brendasbrainstorm.blogspot.com/

Chapter Fourteen
If This is Lucky, I Fold

Carissa Nielsen
Minneapolis, Minnesota

April 6, 2014. I'm thirty years old, a wife, mother, and a highly motivated super human. I have two, maybe three, jobs, I can multitask like a beast, and I have never felt better or more lucky with where I am in life.

April 7, a distracted driver struck my SUV at highway speeds, causing multiple injuries. I was three blocks from home, in an intersection I drove through many times a day, in a neighborhood where I have lived for thirty years, in what was the safest SUV on the market.

And I had the green light.

I opened my eyes to smoke and blood covering everything. I could feel blood rushing down my back, and as I reached for the door handle, my right arm wouldn't move. Thinking my car was on fire, I crawled out and started screaming for someone to help me—I thought I was going to die. A man came to me, and I collapsed into him, begging him to stop all the bleeding. He wrapped a shirt around my head, pushed my blood-gushing hand against my thigh, and covered me with a sweatshirt. We were only ten blocks from the hospital, and I could hear ambulances for what seemed like days, thinking, please hurry...I don't know if I can do this. The man whose shirt and pants I ruined by snuggling my body into his, kept asking me about my family. You're right, I thought, they need me. He keeps chanting, "You're so lucky, you're so lucky."

I could see some hospital staff huddled in the corner, whispering to each other. One of them would look at me and then turn back to the team to whisper some more. I was laying butt naked on the gurney in the ER, bright lights blinding me, my body hurting in 2,873 places, and I was freezing. Finally the nurse who pulled the short straw sulked over to me and said, "We have some bad news. With the laceration on your head, there's a possibility that we will have to shave part of your head." I laughed, "Have you noticed my haircut? It's half-shaved already!" She laughed back in relief, "Don't worry, you'll look great, and you're so lucky!" Damn, my head hurts.

My physical injuries included a broken elbow, broken thumb, and a deep thumb laceration, as well as skull laceration from shattering the window with my head through an airbag. Prescription: surgeries, stitches, casts, slings, physical therapy and pills. I was "lucky"; I looked "great!"

A week later I was attempting to write (now using my left hand), a grocery list for my new helper, a.k.a. husband:
- bread
- OJ
- easy food that can be made 1-handed
- M......

I couldn't figure out what that white stuff was called. You know, you put it on your cereal in the morning. You'd have to leave it open for me in the fridge because now I can't twist anything open. It's from cows. Hmmm...I can spell it: M.I.L.K. Why can't I tell you what it is? Hmm. Weird.

The headaches and insomnia came next. With that came me seeing a neurologist and a new diagnosis: a traumatic brain injury with concussion. According to a Google search, I'm obviously now in a vegetative state, nobody will know what's wrong with me, and there's really no cure. Everything I experience could, or could not be, related to this injury. Boy, am I lucky.

My New Normal...

The last two years have been like an out-of-body experience, like I'm living someone else's life. I'm not the same person, I have a different personality, different interests, different emotions, and different thoughts. I struggle with finding words, mental fog, insomnia, lack of energy, wacky emotional rollercoasters, vertigo, just to name a few things. Gosh, I'm lucky.

I used to be über creative, exciting, personable—I was the fun one! Now it's a daily struggle to make sure I leave the house wearing shoes instead of slippers.

A few notes from my journal:

"I don't recognize my car keys in my purse because they sound different than the keys I had pre-smash. I dig around for an awkwardly long time before I realize they're in there."

"I interrupt people a lot. I realized it's because I have to think so hard about my response (and remember it) that I jump down ahead to spit it out. I'm unintentionally rude now."

"I used to be funny and witty, but now when I try to tell a joke, I say it incorrectly. Or I try to tell a story, and it comes out sounding like a joke because I screwed it up. Now I'm funny because of the random stuff I say, or it's funny that I can't finish a sentence without screwing up. I use humor as a coping mechanism in life, so it doesn't bother me that we laugh at my mushy brain. I just wish my business contacts knew that I had a mushy brain, not just lack of confidence or extreme nervousness."

"Most hilarious thing ever. I'm in the store with a friend, and when a man passes us, I say "Uffdah, too much karaoke!" My friend looks over at me like I'm nuts, and I correct myself. "I mean cologne!" "

So now what?

Sit and be miserable? Once in a while it's okay because you need your lows to appreciate your highs. But I realized that I needed to get off my butt and make this lucky life of mine *count*. I was lucky to be alive. I was lucky to be able to hug my son and husband again. I am lucky that I have slippers to wear on the legs I might not have had.

The more I spoke with other TBI survivors, the less I felt like I was a nutcase or some sort of mad-scientist experiment. What I was going through was very common for TBI survivors, but nobody told me that! I got a "clean bill of health" from doctors, but there was this new mountain to climb…and I finally figured out *that I wasn't alone*.

My husband and I started a purpose-driven company to give back to the TBI Community. We felt an obligation to help others in the places we struggled. We wanted it to be the new normal that TBI survivors talk and sometimes, giggle, about their hurdles, and that they don't feel alone on this journey.

We're survivors.
We tell bad jokes.
We're lucky.
Deal me in.

Carissa Nielsen is an average Minnesotan, wife, mother, and traumatic brain injury survivor. Since her TBI, she and her husband have launched a purpose-driven company, STILL ON™, where they provide free Custom Survival Kits to other TBI survivors and share stories of survivors through their uniquely designed apparel. Carissa is new to being part of the speaker-rotation with the Minnesota Brain Injury Alliance, and she's easy to spot in a crowd with her (usually) blue hair.

Chapter Fifteen
I May Look Fine, But I'm Not

Carol Yost
Bethlehem, Pennsylvania

You must first know the backstory in order to understand where I am today...for concussions are cumulative in their destruction of neurons, and regardless of what anyone tells you, there is no such thing as a mild concussion! The damage may not show itself immediately, and you may not even realize it's there until months later.

My first concussion was suffered in a head-on collision when I was in sixth grade as my forehead broke the entire car windshield. Seatbelts weren't required back then, and we didn't really wear them. The next one occurred a year or two later when I was riding through a neighborhood, hanging onto the side of my father's truck. He wasn't driving fast, but I slipped and fell off, hitting my head on the paved road. The third happened in my thirties when I slipped on ice and hit the back of my head on the sidewalk. I also participated in boxing and mixed martial arts, breaking wood with my head as well as other body parts. There are probably more concussions that I'm not aware of because we just didn't think about hitting your head back then.

And then in August of 2015, I had my fourth concussion now in my fifties. I had always loved to ride bike as a kid. As I aged, life happened and I married and had a daughter. As she grew older, her father and I divorced, and I taught her to ride bike. Unfortunately, she didn't have the love of riding that I did. So being a single mother, riding was put on the back shelf and eventually, I sold my bike as I wasn't using it anymore.

As my daughter grew and moved on with her life, I met someone who reintroduced me to bicycling, and once again I found my love of riding. I started to learn mountain biking and found I loved that as well.

One morning, on a group mountain biking ride, one of the trails had two drops (places where the trail just drops a few feet), and I made it over both drops, but didn't see the tree root at the bottom of the second drop until it was too late. I hit it straight on, and it chalked my front tire causing the bike to stop abruptly. My body flew over the right side of the handlebars and down the embankment, rolling a few times until my helmet-covered head landed on a few rocks. With the exception of the seat and the right hand grip, the bike was fine. I, however, was another story, but I didn't realize it at the time because of adrenaline.

I swore to my friends that I was fine, and that I could ride back to the parking lot once they found and placed the seat back on the bike, as we were almost at the parking lot anyway. Little did I realize that I had received my fourth concussion, and this one was severe. I had broken two ribs and bruised my entire right side. But the physical injuries were nothing compared to the severe concussion. In the parking lot, my friends realized my condition was slipping fast, and rushed me to the hospital.

I don't remember that morning, that day, or the majority of the following four to six weeks. I have only bits and pieces of that time frame, and my life has been a nightmare since. I couldn't do things that had come naturally to me prior to the crash. Walking was a major task as my balance was like someone who had way too much to drink, and staggering was the best I could do. I couldn't read, watch TV, and even talking was an issue because the words wouldn't leave my brain to come out of my mouth.

The hospital ordered physical and occupational therapy, which started within a week of my release from the hospital. I had to live with my sister because she has a one-level ranch house and I have a two-story home. The hospital wouldn't release me otherwise for fear of me falling again. My sister was an angel taking care of me. Looking back, we scheduled the appointments for the morning, because that's when I was at my best. As the day progressed, I became worn out. I took lots of naps, and had trouble remembering everything and anything. We shouldn't have scheduled my appointments for when I was at my best—this meant that doctors and therapists saw me at my best, and never at my worst. After six weeks, I returned to my own home.

The doctors released me to go back to work part-time just over two months after my accident, with no restrictions except I was limited to no more than four hours of work per day. The exam that released me to return to work was simply whether I stand with my eyes closed without wobbling, and how did I feel? Well, I felt like Wonder Woman!! Of course, this was compared to how I felt right after my fourth concussion.

My return to work lasted seven days. I worked Monday and Tuesday, and these days were not terrible, but by Wednesday, people started to realize I had returned to work, and they came and asked me to do work. Even though I would explain that I was only back part-time, they would still say, "Well, I need this." This was always preceded or followed by, "You look great!" When I left work on Wednesday, once home, I went straight to bed. This same thing happened on Thursday and Friday. I slept all weekend, rising only to eat and go to the bathroom. I returned to work Monday and Tuesday for four hours each day, but by the time I left work on Tuesday, I was so mentally toasted that I could not function, and had relapsed back to where I was shortly after the accident.

A friend forced me to call my doctor, who pulled me from work immediately. When I saw the doctor the following week, I was referred to a neurologist who ordered further occupational and physical therapy. I used up all of the visits the insurance company would allow, but still had issues. Luckily it was almost the end of the calendar year, and new visits would kick in as of January 1, so we held off until the new year.

During the intake exam at occupational therapy in the new year, the intern performing it noticed a twitch in my eye. The therapist confirmed this, and a few weeks later when it hadn't gone away, she referred me to a neurological ophthalmologist. He confirmed a blind spot existed in my left eye caused by repeated concussions. I didn't even know that I had it because my right eye picks up the balance of the required vision, as long as both eyes are open. He also discovered issues with my ability to track/read across a page and maintain my place. I began 24 weeks of vision therapy. The simplest of tasks were so very difficult to do, but I had to master them before moving on to harder tasks. We worked on only one eye at a time to strengthen each eye individually. Once we accomplished that, we could move on to working both eyes together.

All this time, friends and people in general looked at me and said, "You don't look like anything is wrong." Well, I'd love for them to live for just a few hours inside my head. I've considered suicide because it's just so tough, but then I think how many others have it so much worse than me.

The worst part is when the medical community doesn't believe you or makes light of what you are going through.

Every single visit, my occupational therapist kept triggering something so that my symptoms occurred. They got worse and worse each time; it was as if it was a challenge to her. And then she would belittle what I was feeling. My insurance company would approve only twelve visits, so my occupational therapy ended without resolution of my issues.

My neurologist told my long-term disability insurance that there was nothing wrong with me neurologically–that I was simply suffering from headaches. This was news to me because she had never even discussed that with me. This, of course, cut off my income.

Appealing to the disability insurance, filing for Social Security Disability, losing my job and my medical insurance, not knowing where to turn, and having no one to help me navigate these areas, all left me tired and worn out. No one understands, and no one knows what to do, and besides, you "look fine," so what's the problem?

Luckily, I've been able to find a few folks that do care and are pointing me in the right direction. I've been scheduled for a neurological psych exam that will help determine the next step.

It's a sad state of affairs. We know so much and yet, so little about our brains. The medical field doesn't seem to care enough to dig deeper to support us. The problem is that we are suffering, and we should be getting support and help.

Carol is an unemployed brain injury survivor striving to get her life back as much as possible. She's a fighter, not giving up even though some doctors have shaken her off, which is common for most survivors. She has since found her team members who know what to do, and is working hard on her therapy and fighting off the depression that ensues after such an injury.

Chapter Sixteen
Sharing Hard-Earned Advice

Caroline Charpentier
Québec, Canada

In 2012, time stopped—because I began a new relationship with my TBI/concussion.

Before this event, I knew very little about TBI/concussions. I knew as much about it as I knew about Mount Everest. Now, *I'm climbing this mountain.*

TBI/concussion has big implications. If you're dealing now with this reality, I understand. If you feel you're lost, that's normal.

Many symptoms I don't like come with TBI/concussion. With time, I became more used to them. They are like my new housemate. I know, with time, it's important to try to learn how to deal with them each day. Just try! This is why I try to call my TBI/concussion more like a housemate than an enemy. I think it's more helpful to deal with him than to always be angry at him. What do you think about that?

The recovery process is like a rollercoaster, and sometimes I would want the ride to slow down or stop completely. "Okay, we are closing this attraction today and for the rest of the summer. See you next season!" But, it's not that easy with a TBI/concussion.

I want to encourage you in this hard moment. Here are some thoughts to remember that help me when time is rough:

- It's okay…you can be angry about this situation.

- It's okay if you cry.

- Show, talk about, or write down your emotions, it's important…and it helps.

- Visit and participate in the many supporter groups on Facebook or Twitter because it can help us. We are not alone.

- Live more "one day at a time." It's more helpful than worrying about what's coming in two months.

- Learn your limits. Your body is talking to you.

- Allow some time to rest during the day.

- Divide your activities into steps rather than trying to do everything in one shot.

- Do something you like: reading, watching funny videos, paint, see a friend.

- Don't be shy to tell others how your feel, and reach out for help when you need it

- Be kind to yourself. Be smart with yourself. Be with yourself like you are with your best friend.

- Keep moving at your own pace and at your rhythm, according to your symptoms.

- Remember: "Don't give up." Don't give up, please. Don't.

Author Mary Anne Radmacher, wrote: "Courage does not always roar. Sometimes courage is the quiet voice at the end of the day saying, 'I will try again tomorrow." Yes, because some days are really tough, and you can wait until tomorrow for the next step.

With all these events in my life, now I see life differently. I enjoy the present moments more. Now I know life is fragile…and I must take care of it. I see TBI/concussion like the vegetation after a forest fire. The vegetation regenerates again, after a while, like my brain, like my life. Or like the flower that grows in the middle of the street while we might think it is impossible that vegetation can grow there. I cling to these examples because they help keep me being hopeful.

Finally, the goal is not to be at the top of the Everest Mount. The goal is simply to climb, make own way—and whatever the result is, we are a winner *because we are of one those survivors.*

Caroline Charpentier is a person who lives with the reality of repetitive concussions. She is a psychoeducator. Each time she can, she likes to speak and write about this subject to raise awareness. She knows the real face of this injury, and she wants to help others.

Chapter Seventeen
The Day I Chose Life

Cat Castellanos
Washington, DC

I'm not your typical TBI patient, if there is such a thing. There was no crash car, no IED, no blow to the head. But boy, was I hit.

In 2005, when I was 18 years old, I arrived in the ER screaming in pain. I had bacterial meningitis, a disease that will kill in four hours.

The inflammation caused the equivalent of a TBI. It's hard to explain to other people about a brain injury created by your own body. No, there was no trauma if you define it by "impact," but the consequences were traumatic in every sense of the word.

You see I spent a decade suffering from a brain injury I didn't know I had. In my naivety, I assumed that since my body had healed, my brain had as well. After a year in and out of the hospital and another year in recovery, I began to take on the world as I had always intended: College, relationships, jobs, and the typical bacchanalia required of those in their twenties.

Had you met me, you would have met the superlative version; the social, outgoing, determined Cat. But the real me woke up thinking, "What do I have to do to get back to bed?" I was constantly exhausted, yet my limbs were all in place and my skin remained unmarred—so I thought the fatigue, anxiety, and mental fog, "must be my own weakness."

Most of our lives are defined by certain moments, and I had one such juncture during my first year in college. From my bed, I reached over to grab my phone and saw eight missed messages from friends wondering whether I wanted to join them for a movie, for dinner at the dining hall, for a drink at the bar, to go over study notes, for life. Despite having a full night of rest, I had slept through an entire afternoon and evening's worth of activities, and I was still tired. I had once again missed the day.

That day is what I refer to as "The Day I Chose Life." I decided that I could sleep the rest of my life away, or I could get up and push. I resigned myself to the fact that my life would be one of self-management. And so I drank coffee, took stimulants, and congratulated myself when I was able to ignore the voice in my head that told me to go back to bed.

I pushed until I became a graduate, a girlfriend, and finally, a writer. At one point I was hired to do a story on veterans with PTSD. Despite hours of interviews and days of editing, I had become so detached that *I failed to recognize any of the symptoms in myself.*

It's not that I didn't know something was wrong. I just thought it was me, that my depression was a weakness, not the result of a brain injury. I sought help from traditional sources, but medications and psychiatrists did nothing to fix the underlying problem. Years passed as I band-aided my way through life, until a chance situation changed everything.

I shouldn't have been there in the first place. The first time I missed the conference was due to an urgent trip home to see my neurologist, who told me my symptoms were the equivalent of PTSD. Still struggling two months later, I almost canceled on the conference again, but in classic fashion, pushed myself to go. I'm glad I did. I happened upon a presentation about the treatment of veterans and autism using a version of transcranial magnetic stimulation (TMS), a non-invasive treatment to activate "sleeping" neurons in the brain.

Fast forward a year, and now after 200 treatments, I'm a new person. I'm awake during the day and asleep at night. I have energy. My mind is clearer. Most of all, I'm one person, not two.

The hardest part of was thinking I was crazy for all those years—that it was my weakness, my fault, not my brain injury. The saddest part? I had become resigned to think of myself as broken and beyond help.

After treatment, I began researching neuroplasticity, the idea that your brain has a remarkable ability to evolve and grow, regardless of your age, condition, or mental capacity.

It's now my life's mission to experiment with everything from magnetic stimulation to meditation and MDMA-assisted psychotherapy to find out how to improve my stamina, focus, and mood—and then bring that information to others.

I want people to know that it's never too late. You can improve, even ten years down the line.

Cat Castellanos works with the relentlessly ambitious, offering customized, science-based coaching programs for improved sleep, memory, focus, and productivity.

Chapter Eighteen
One Woman, One Trike, 5,390 Miles

Catherine Brubaker
Tempe, Arizona

I had reached a management level in the financial services industry while achieving my M.S. in Organizational Leadership. My undergrad was in Psychology. In 2010, I came very close to losing my life due to a violent criminal assault. The lack of oxygen and no respiratory support overnight left me with a *diffused axonal anoxic brain injury*. As a result of my injuries, my heart began to fail, and I developed post-concussive syndrome.

It was like a fire came into my life and destroyed everything, and I was left with some structure and ashes. I didn't know it could happen to me. I lost the ability to walk and communicate. Performance testing revealed grade school-level functioning—after having the responsibilities of writing Individualized Educational Plans (IEP) for children with intellectual disabilities early in my career.

I felt like I fell into a black hole, without any explanation or anyone noticing. I slept or was zoned out most of the time. I began a very long road of rehabilitation.

While riding home after a post-op visit because I had just received a pacemaker, I was in a serious motor vehicle accident as a passenger, resulting in complicating my post-concussive syndrome. I was sent back to square one. My rehabilitation required hospitalization, inpatient, outpatient and a day program, which was a very lengthy process. As a result of my traumatic brain injuries, my autonomic system is damaged, my heart began to fail, and I have challenges with temperature control, respiration, digestion, and blood pressure. I was diagnosed with a form of dysautonomia, severe postural orthostatic tachycardia (P.O.T.S.), which causes blood to pool in my abdomen and legs. Standing for any length of time is difficult, but exercising helps.

As a result, I received a pacemaker. Symptoms are difficult to manage, and I found the ER staff has little understanding of it. I exercise to increase blood flow and increase circulation, and I frequently wear tight-fitting compression clothing to combat these symptoms. From time to time, I have to go to the hospital to receive IV hydration, as my body struggles with efficiency in managing electrolytes.

Even though I struggle, often severely, I am determined to recover, find answers and give hope to others along this bittersweet journey. It can have a silver lining, and we have the potential to write our own story on our road to recovery.

In 2014, I was the first woman in history to cross the United States on a recumbent trike, after having had two traumatic brain injuries. I dipped my tire in the ocean in Washington, and five months later, arrived in Key West, Florida, where I celebrated my journey of 5390 miles by dipping my tire in the Atlantic Ocean.

This had been an introspective journey of a lifetime, and it allowed me to rise from the ashes. My trip was possible because of the support of members of my community. I learned that I could ride across the country, but my invisible challenges still made it difficult for others to understand my TBI. Often I am judged by my appearance rather than my ability—and this helped me find my passion, dig deep for my voice, and find a way to contribute in a productive and meaningful way. I found that I was not alone and that others had similar challenges, some even more severe, which gave me a sense of gratitude and perspective—and that perspective changed everything.

For that reason, I founded Hope For Trauma, a non-profit 501(3) c with the vision of being an advocate in a national conversation about the challenges faced by brain injury survivors and their families. I am currently doing that through HOPE TV, and by participating on the Brain Injury Association of America Advisory Council. The mission is to provide adaptive cycling and other equipment directly to those traumatic brain injury (TBI) survivors. I travel the country, and through speaking engagements, I share my very personal and powerful story of hope, as well as capture other stories to bridge the gap of fear and misunderstanding.

In 2016, I was awarded the Trailblazer Award from The Brain Injury Alliance of Arizona (BIAAZ) for my work with TBI survivors. Mayor Mark Mitchell, City of Tempe, Arizona, presented me with the 2016 Tempe Bike Hero award. Congresswoman Kyrsten Sinema wrote a letter of recognition for my achievements and continued work. I was recently nominated for the Blue Cross Blue Shield Hometown Hero, I was recognized on center court at the Phoenix Mercury 2016, and was recently asked to testify in front of city council on bike paths and the access for adaptive cycles for the disabled community.

I believe that as a community, survivor advocates can leave the greatest legacy of hope.

Catherine Brubaker, M.S.L., Executive Director of Hope For Trauma, is the first woman in history to cross the United States on an adaptive cycle after she had suffered two brain injuries. She is a tireless advocate for brain injury awareness, serving on the Brain Injury Association of America's Advisory Council. www.hopefortrauma.org

Chapter Nineteen
Surviving and Thriving

Cathy Stewart
Tucson, Arizona

You may wonder about how I can write so well. There's a different part of your brain that's accessed when you write, versus when you talk. My conversations are not the same. I have a hard time with things like word retrieval, losing my train of thought, and expressing myself verbally. I don't think you could tell by my writing that I have a TBI.

So here's a very small bit of how I acquired my TBI in 2004. It was a normal workday for me. Heading out to see my clients, I worked as an RN care manager for at-risk seniors living with dementia. Little did I know how much this day would change me forever.

Thankfully I don't have any memories of the accident. I don't have to experience living over and over in my mind how a semi-truck rear-ended me. All I know is what I remember being told by my attorney, who had the accident scene recreated for my personal injury law suit.

Traveling 65 mph while looking down at his map, this rookie driver of only two weeks looked up to see my van's brake lights lit up. There's a lot more involved in this situation, but I'll leave out those details. He rear-ended my car, pushing me into another vehicle, and then I went flying end over end, landing on the roadside. This was all witnessed by Colorado highway department workers. At the deposition, one of them said watching this was better than any action movie he'd seen. I had *no memories* of that happening.

I was told that I was awake when I arrived in the emergency room. I had a subarachnoid hemorrhage along with traumatic brain injury, bone contusions, and a major shoulder injury. Very thankfully, I didn't require surgery.

After being in a coma for four days, I started responding. I was totally confused. I couldn't see because of double vision, my balance was really bad, I was in pain because of my other injuries and also because of nerve damage in my face. I couldn't think. My brain was so slow. And all I could do was sleep.

I was sent home within a couple days of when I started responding. It took a really good team of rehab pros to get me going on my long road of starting my life again as a different person. Even though there wasn't a rehab facility in the area where I lived, my doctor was able to surround me with what I needed to work at recovering my lost abilities.

At that time, my then-husband was away a lot for his sales job, and we had two elementary-age children and one ninth-grader at home.

With years of hard work, I'm now functioning, successfully living on my own, driving again, even on interstates. These things happened many years down the road because my persistence kept me trying, and I finally succeeded.

Currently, I'm 12 years out from my injuries. It's been a long haul, kind of like a marathon maybe. I'm thankful and filled with gratitude every day that I wake to my doggy's kisses. Stay strong, love yourself, advocate for yourself, enjoy the small things, use positive self-talk and remember, *a nap will help.*

Not just a survivor, Cathy has been living her life to the fullest following her severe TBI. In her previous life, she was a high-functioning, multitasking registered nurse for 25 years, and Mom to three much-loved children. Cathy now calls Tucson, Arizona home.

Chapter Twenty
Always a Driven Person

Christelle Kay Harris
Monterey, California

I was always driven. My mother once told me that I was always upset because I didn't "know enough." This must have been why I decided to join the military on August 20, 2001, twelve days before the September 11th terror attack. I served eight years as an aircraft mechanic, and enjoyed every moment of it.

I didn't join the military to serve my country; I'm not that patriotic. I joined so I could go to college and afford it. I was in a Master's degree program to become a Clinical Mental Health Counselor when it happened. I was in the bike lane, riding my bright orange beach cruiser bicycle home from the public library after doing my homework, I had just stopped at the appropriate stop sign, and then it happened. A man in an old white Nissan Sentra ran his stop sign. He was text messaging, and didn't look up—he just hit me.

I'll be frank; I don't remember him hitting me. The police said that I went backwards, head first through his windshield and "damaged his windshield." There was nothing in the initial police report about his windshield causing a cone fracture to my skull, and subdural hematoma in my occipital, parietal and temporal lobes. The police report never mentioned that I was immediately admitted to the University of Utah Neural Critical Care Unit.

My damaged brain failed to remember the first four days I spent in the Neural Critical Care Unit. When I woke up, I had no recollection of the horrors I had experienced, nor any idea of what I would experience. My mother had flown from California to Utah the moment she found out, and she was in the room when I woke up. She announced to me, along with my three nurses, a neurosurgeon and a neurologist that I had literally *become my worst nightmare*, like the creature in Franz Kafka's "Metamorphosis." I was now the opposite of what I had worked my whole life to become. I was unable to move my own body (called proprioception), unable to speak (verbal aphasia) and unable to express emotions, except anger.

I had no choice but to begin my journey out into the world again, but as a different person.

After leaving the hospital, my family decided that I deserved a nice dinner out in a restaurant. I notoriously loved restaurants, until now. The restaurant was packed with innocent people carrying on with their normal lives. They were talking, tending to their crying babies, having dates, enjoying being out with their children, and eating with utensils on hard plates. Just normal, everyday things—unless you have a traumatic brain injury.

I was immediately introduced to my brain's new reality. The smallest sounds radiated pain through my head and body, and I was overwhelmed by every word people spoke around me. Life had become like a broad-stroke painting, consisting of neon, glow-in-the-dark colors. Every word, sound and sight was like a physical assault. In this situation, one can quickly become very angry because of pain, confusion and lack of understanding—and I did. This hypersensitivity still exists three years later.

If you know traumatic brain injury, you know healing is measured in years, and often a person never returns to his or her normal self. I'm not going to hash out what my healing process took and is taking. I'll just say this: it is still taking a lot of my resilience, my energy, my intellect, and all of my human abilities three years later.

Ironically, it is not having a traumatic brain injury that affects my life as much anymore—it is *the social injustice* I will forever incur.

The man who hit me got only a $90 traffic ticket, while I lost my job as a University counselor, had to leave graduate school, and am still struggling with $300,000 in medical bills. This man hit me in a no-fault state, and is therefore not responsible for the repercussions of his negligence. Anyone in this situation would have been mad. Driven by the anger that welled up inside me, I took action.

When my brain had healed enough to conceive of what the world needed, and I had enough understanding to research the epidemic of traumatic brain injury—2.5 million people a year acquire a brain injury, and not all of them live. Knowing all this, I decided the best path for everyone experiencing the fear, hopelessness, and relentless healing process of a TBI, was to make a documentary. I decided to illustrate and bring to life the reality of what a person with a TBI goes through, both physically and socially. So, two years into the process of healing, I bought a camera, and then contacted two friends, one who is a director and one with a sound stage, and I started recording everything. I contacted public figures that had appropriate things to say about social justice, I recorded myself weeping on the phone with officials who told me that legally it was hopeless. I also showed the fifth wheel RV I am now living in, as well as the training of my service animal. Everything.

One might think that this seemingly painstaking process would be near impossible, or create more anger, more hopelessness or worse, cause a person with a TBI to give up completely. I'm happy to report that recording everything and everyone brought new hope and insight to the *new normal* of my life after traumatic brain injury. Life through a lens allows you to see things in detailed perspective. I began to notice how grateful I was for the beautiful colors of my service animal's fur, and her soulful eyes. I noticed the clearness of the water I drank. I allowed myself to feel a deep gratitude for the people who had both helped me, and those who had taught me. I watched myself laughing, and trying to first walk, then run, do yoga, climb, surf and ski again.

I have discovered that helping others is one of the most beautiful things any human being can do, and I have kept my head down and have been pushing ever since. I have just re-enrolled in school in order to finish my internships and fulfill my dream of counseling people in need of help and advocacy.

The first thing every single person who acquires a brain injury is going to hear out of my mouth is "You are *not alone.*"

Christelle is a surfer, road bike rider, and lover of our precious Earth. She is filming a documentary about traumatic brain injury, and invisible disabilities. She holds a Master's degree in clinical counseling, and hopes to help those with disabilities once she gains her license.

Chapter Twenty-One
Taking Control of My New Normal

Courtney G. Lee
Sacramento, California

The doctor shrugged and shook his head dismissively. "It's been two years, so you shouldn't waste your time on therapy. It's not going to get any better." He collected his chart and pen from the table where he laid them about five minutes earlier when he walked into the examination room and met me for the first time. "Okay?"

My polite smile and nod betrayed the fact that my heart had fallen into my stomach. "Okay. Thank you!" I left the office, and tried not to let the other people in the parking lot see my tears.

It wasn't so much this doctor's words that shattered my soul. He does not know me, and he isn't even specialized in neuroscience; he was acting as a middleman—and in this case, a barrier—before I could be referred to that specialist (ah, the wonderful health care system). It wasn't his words; it was the quiet, nagging voice in the back of my head that they confirmed.

It *had* been two years since my cycling accident in 2014. I am a professor, and on that beautiful May morning I was grading final exam papers at home. I decided to take a break and do something outside to clear my head. My husband, Scott, was out on a long bike ride and would be on his way home, so I pulled my own bike out of the garage, and thankfully strapped my helmet on tightly like I always did. I encountered Scott on the bike path as planned and turned around to ride the rest of the way back with him. I remember how perfect the day was: bright and clear, not too hot, not too windy.

The next thing I remember is lying in my bed at home, with Scott telling me that I could not go to work. My head was anything but clear.

What happened in between those two memories included me losing control of my bicycle—we're still not entirely sure how, but Scott suspects it may have been related to the tire pressure—and me being projected off the front at sixteen miles per hour onto the pavement, absorbing the full impact with my head. He thought I was dead until I started making incomprehensible noises while he held me still and waited for the ambulance. At the hospital, social workers sat with him, discussing grief, and what might happen if I didn't make it.

Fortunately I did pull through somehow, and based on what Scott tells me, I am infinitely grateful to have no recollection of the accident or my time in the ICU with its needles, tubes, tests, and various associated indignities. I do have a single dim, blessedly brief memory of a neck brace that could have doubled as a medieval torture device, and of throwing up while wearing it. I guess I hate vomiting so much that even a concussion and drugs couldn't block that out. I must confess that I feel a little cheated that I do not remember the ambulance ride, though. Apparently they used the sirens and blew through intersections and everything. Since I'm too old now to realize my erstwhile dream of rock stardom, that's probably the closest I will get to have a police escort, and I didn't even get to enjoy it.

Once I was home again after four days in the hospital, I was glad to experience what felt like rapid progress for the first six months or so. My left eye remained closed for most of that time, but I celebrated little victories, like when I made it through at least half of a sentence before forgetting the rest of what I wanted to say, when I stood up in the shower for the first time, or when I successfully pulled on my jeans while standing up and not holding onto anything. When my left eye finally started to open, I wore a pirate patch (literally, I bought it at a costume shop), because my left eye looked far to the left, regardless of where my right eye focused.

Cognitively, today my aphasia (not being able to find the words I want to say) has lessened to the point that most people do not notice it unless I point it out. My mood swings are not as severe, including the bouts of unprompted and uncontrollable laughter, which I actually kind of miss. My headaches continue, but are less debilitating, or perhaps I just have grown used to them. I returned to work, and although it was challenging, I adapted and generally feel like I have fallen back into place.

I attribute these developments to a few things, like:
- Building neuroplasticity by playing brain games each day and revisiting rusty old skills, like my high school Spanish training or playing the guitar;
- Reading as much as I can, beginning with short ads and slowly working up to books;
- Meeting with a tremendous speech therapist that also introduced me to the benefits of mindfulness and meditation (thank you, Renee!); and
- Doing exercise, like yoga and walking.

But most of all, I credit my husband. From the first seconds after impact to today, he has been nothing but patient, kind, understanding, and supportive, holding me up both figuratively and literally. I know this has been as hard for him as it has been for me, if not harder, and I never take for granted how incredibly fortunate I am to have him in my life.

Physically, progress has been more sluggish. I stopped using my pirate patch, but my left eye still does not track with the right, and it is more heavy-lidded. I often joke that I could be a stand-in for Sloth from "The Goonies" movie, although Scott does not share my amusement. As a result of my injuries, I see double in the majority of my field of vision, and I use a cane for stability. I am so grateful to be able to walk at all, but even though my cane is painted with butterflies, and we decorate it with battery-operated lights during the holidays, using a cane really isn't much fun. I will admit that it's pretty terrific at airports, however; it's surprisingly satisfying to sit quietly, and then board the plane in front of the people who have stood smugly in the first-class line for an hour, just so everyone else can see how important they are. Despite that, I've been trying to use it less, often carrying a retractable hiking stick instead that I can extend if needed.

It was easy to stay positive when I could see little improvements each day or week, but now my sails feel limp, leaving me mired in what appear to be stagnant waters with no suggestion of a breeze on the horizon. I hadn't realized how much ostensibly generic affirmations of recovery buoyed my spirits, especially from medical professionals: "Every brain injury is different." "Recovery takes time." "You've made great strides." "Be patient." At the doctor's office on that day mentioned above, I hoped that he might at least repeat those encouraging sentiments. Instead, he confirmed what has terrified me for so long: *that this is it, and things are as good as they are going to get.*

Of course I appreciate his honesty, if that's what it was, and his comments did cause me to shift my focus. I realized that I had been waiting to try to do certain things until I returned to my pre-accident state; for example, I thought, "Once I stop seeing double, I can stop using this cane." Now, instead of waiting, I am trying to adjust to what could be *my new normal*: "I might be able to see straight again one day, but either way I'm going to try to walk across campus without extending my cane today." I do not think there is anything wrong or embarrassing about using a cane; it just gets in my way, and I would like to stop using it if I can. I also rode a bicycle again last month; it was for only a few hundred feet on a road in a cemetery with no traffic, but I didn't panic or fall, so I classify it as a success.

No matter what, I will not allow that doctor's—or anyone else's—undiplomatic comments and insensitive demeanor to pull me into pessimism and depression. I will take his and any other negative comments I encounter along the way, turn them around, and use them to fuel more positive change. I will work with what I have to accomplish as much as I can, which may be more than I'm told I will be able to do. I just heard a story from someone whose doctor told him he would never run again, but twenty-two marathons and four Ironman triathlons later, he begs to differ. There are thousands of stories like that, and I will write my own to add to the list.

I encourage anyone struggling with TBI recovery to add his or her own story, too, even though it may take years to write. Hold on to those standard encouraging affirmations, and use any negative comments to spur you onward, whether it's to prove them wrong or to help you adjust your own perspective, because every head injury *is* different, and recovery *does* take time. Surround yourself with love and support, remind yourself of how far you've come, celebrate victories large and small, and take the time you need to mold your new normal into something that might be even better than the old one.

Courtney G. Lee suffered a TBI in a 2014 cycling crash that also affected her third cranial nerve, causing what appears to be permanent double vision (she is thankful that her helmet saved her life). She continues to work on improving her cognitive skills and balance, and generally adjusting to her "new normal" while fulfilling her duties as a law professor. When not working, she enjoys spending time with her magnificent husband and their cats.

Chapter Twenty-Two
A Second Can Change Your Life Forever

Cyndi Syverson
Blaine, Minnesota

On Jan. 13, 2015 at 6:15 pm, I was playing with my grandchildren, age three, and age one. We were waiting for their mom, Amy, our oldest daughter, to pick them up on her way home from work. When the phone rang, something told me it wasn't good. The caller said Amy was in a severe car accident, and was unconscious at the scene. I called Amy's husband, Michael, and told him what happened and to meet the ambulance at the hospital.

The last year and a half of our lives has been a nightmare...and I keep hoping I can wake up. A traumatic brain injury doesn't just happen to the victim, it happens to the entire family. Amy and her two children moved into our home for six months because Amy was unable to take care of the kids, let alone herself. Michael came over every night for dinner and to put the kids to bed, and then drove 21 miles north to their home to take care of the dog and other things.

Amy went through two TBI programs at two major Twin City Hospitals. Amy said when she was unconscious she had seen Jesus at the Gates of Heaven with his arms open wide to her.

My new life became driving Amy to daily doctor appointments plus physical, occupational and speech therapy. I couldn't even begin to count how many trips to the hospital/emergency room we had her first year. After six months, we were able to move Amy and the kids back to their home in Oak Grove where they stayed four days a week, and at our house three days a week. I went to their house on the days they are there, staying until Michael comes home from work.

Amy had total double-blurred vision the first year post-TBI. She now has glasses that are tinted yellow due to her light sensitivity, and the glasses have multiple prisms that are taped off by her nosepiece. This is needed, due to her poor peripheral vision. She has been nauseated due to the vision problems 24/7 since the accident. She takes antiemetic medications around the clock, with little relief of the nausea. I've had to become like a pharmacist, as Amy is on so many meds that change frequently. She is very drug sensitive, and has many bad side effects, causing the need for frequent dose and med changes.

People say… well, at least her kids are young, and it doesn't affect them… but that is definitely not true. Anyone who knows those two children can see what it's done to their life. First of all, the first six months they had many different babysitters. Many of the people were friends volunteering their time to help us out. The kids had never met most of them, and never knew who would be there when they got up from their naps. Her daughter became very clingy and wanted to be at her mom's side, and didn't want her to leave her sight. She is so used to others taking care of her and her needs, that to this day she has trouble listening to her mom and following her direction. She has been going to therapy for the last six months, in order to understand what life is like with her mom now, the way she is.

Amy has short-term memory loss, and she tires and fatigues easily. She is severely depressed, trying to accept *who the new Amy is*. Luckily we recently found her a great therapist who she meets with weekly. She has *very high* anxiety, and can go from a 1 to 10 plus in 1.2 seconds. Any change in her normal routine, or getting ready for an appointment or outing, is sure to send her to a 10-plus. It is hard not to get mad at her, and I have had to bite my tongue several times a day. *I can't imagine what it's like to live one day in her life.*

Then to top it off, their son has been diagnosed with low-spectrum autism. He is *very* active, and everything has to be his way. He gets private occupational therapy and speech twice a week, and once a week from the school district. So we get to add that to our bag of tricks. He is definitely a momma's boy. He also gets very upset with any change in his routine, and is very frightened of strangers.

Michael comes home after working ten-hour days, and has to take over all the responsibilities of taking care of his family. He never complains; he just does what he has to do to keep his family going. Their family life has totally changed, as before the accident, they were always on the go, hiking, biking, or exploring new things.

It's hard for people to understand what life is really like for Amy. If you look at her, she looks like a normal 29-year-old, with tinted, funky-looking glasses. Most people don't understand what a TBI really is, and thus think that she is lazy and doesn't want to go back to work. Believe me, she would go back to work in a heartbeat if she could.

It hurts Amy terribly to hear hurtful comments from others.

To tell you the truth I didn't know a lot about TBIs myself until January 13, 2015. Since then I've learned more than I ever wanted to know, and truly feel I could teach a class to the public to better inform them what a TBI is, what it can do to the victim, and what it can do to the victim's family.

Watching what my daughter Amy has gone through the last year and a half of her life totally breaks my heart, day after day. She will never be the same wife, mom, daughter or sister she was before the accident. We all thank God daily for letting her stay in our lives, as we know how close we came to losing her that day. Life is a gift we must cherish every day. You never know from one second to the next what challenges you will be handed. Just remember all things happen for a reason, and through God, all things are possible.

Cyndi is the mother of 29-year-old Amy Lockman, who suffered a TBI after a car accident on January 13, 2015. Amy and Michael have two children, age three and five. Sadly, a TBI involves the entire family.

Chapter Twenty-Three
C'est la Vie

Danielle Houston Karst
Burke, Virginia

Sometimes life sucks, and circumstances suck, but that's life. There's nothing else you can say or do about it. I, of all people, think I know that best. When life gives you lemons, make lemonade. Sigh.

In 1997, there was an awful car accident between a Jeep Cherokee and another car driven by a young guy, speeding around a corner. The young girl in the Jeep was driving a friend home after a cheerleading performance. The car accident happened on the first Saturday morning after the new school year had started.

I'm the 16-year-old girl in the Jeep, the young traumatic brain injury survivor. The accident put me in a comatose state from which I woke up 2½ months later, right before Thanksgiving.

I turned my car left, past a lane of oncoming traffic when another car came around the corner and didn't see me in time. I was told the 19-year-old driver slammed into the driver's side and flipped my Jeep over. I had to be cut from the car by the "jaws of life." However, I don't remember because I was unconscious upon impact. It was only 10:30 in the morning, but I do remember some things that already happened that day. I remember that the grass was wet with the early morning dew, and the girls who were on the top for the stunts had to have the bottoms of their shoes towel dried, and then be carried around by other cheerleaders. When my friend asked for a ride home, I remembered saying that I wasn't allowed to drive with other people in the car yet. I changed my mind, and almost insisted on driving her home; I was still excited I could drive, and wanted to show her that I can. I remember putting on my seatbelt.

After being in the ICU for nearly a month, I was transported to Kluge's Children's Rehabilitation Center in Charlottesville, Virginia. My parents did not know what to think—the doctors and specialists were telling them everything from: I'd never wake up, if I did, I'd be in a vegetative state, to I'd be totally fine. No one knows what to say with a brain injury because the brain is so complex.

Therapy at the hospital would go on all day. I would have physical, occupational, and speech therapy, as well as counseling with a social worker, and school therapy, where we would work on basic writing, and holding a pencil. Every day I would participate in aquatic therapy, even while I was in a semi-comatose state. I could still walk holding onto two people, and the movements of the water would be very helpful in regaining my equilibrium. In water, a person is weightless, and I worked on the mechanics and the structure of walking—butt in, lift the feet and push the chest forward. I was using a wheelchair to get around between therapy sessions in the hospital. In physical therapy I was working on stepping, with my heels then my toes, but that never worked because I would always tiptoe around at first anyway.

A few months later I watched a video of my first attempt at walking, and was amazed at how long it took me to walk down the hallway. In physical therapy I would use a standing box to get my weight spread more evenly onto my heels. The standing box is a podium on a platform that was stood on. There is a condition informally called "drop-toe" or foot drop that happens to people who are unconscious a long time, and thus are not walking or flexing their feet so the muscles relax and the foot points forward, almost on tiptoes. I wore casts on my feet/legs to try to keep the feet flexed, and after I "woke up," I worked on shifting my weight to my heels.

In occupational therapy, while I was still in a coma, the therapist was working on my senses, like olfactory/smell by sticking strong smelling herbs in my face. They said I scrunched up my nose and made faces. In my speech therapy we would work on breath control, enunciating and memory. The therapist held up pictures, like of the Washington monument, and I answered "the big pencil." She shook her head no, and my mom was cracking up in the background saying, "No, that's what she's always called it." I was shown other pictures of common items, and got a lot of them correct, could describe them, but could not think of the word. The speech and language pathologist showed me a picture of Princess Diana soon after I came out of my coma. I identified her correctly, and said, "But isn't she dead?" Her car accident had made news only a few weeks before mine. My memory was very selective, remembering some events, but not others.

Even though life continued for all of my classmates, they hadn't forgotten me. *All* my friends were at Fairfax Hospital when I was in the ICU, and a lot of my friends came to visit me in the rehab hospital in Charlottesville. This included friends from my cheerleading all-star squad, the boys that were on the baseball team at my high school and my closest friend who was the maid of honor at my wedding 10 years later, so my hospital room was the place to be on the weekends. Just kidding, but I did get a lot of visitors. My hospital room was covered with cards and stuffed animals, plus both of my cheerleading squads made me get-well banners.

I "woke up" one day while my dad was helping me with dinner. I had a gastrointestinal tube in my stomach to give me medication and food, but the nurses were working on getting me to ingest food orally. Dad must have looked the other way, or got up without putting up the railing on the side of my bed, and a split second later, I had rolled onto the floor, bumping my head. He hugged me close, and apologized again and again.

I think that fall must have knocked some sense into me, because I remember everything from that day forward. It must have been a Saturday, because Dad was with me. He switched off with Mom, who had taken a leave of absence from work to stay with me during the workweek, while Dad would be at home working and staying with my brother. On Sunday my brother traveled up with Mom to the hospital. When he walked in, I just laughed and laughed. I swore that it wasn't really my brother, because he was so big and tall. I asked him what grade he was in (eighth), his age (13), and when he told me this, I burst out laughing again because I remembered him as a short little blond, but his hair had turned a golden brown as he had gotten older. I believed he was my brother, but found the whole situation hilarious.

I was allowed a home pass for Christmas, because I had been one of the patients with the longest stay. It was great being at home for Christmas that year. Our family did what we always do—have a "German Weinachten" over at my grandmother's, attending a church service, dinner and opening presents from Oma and Uncle Pat, and then doing the whole traditional Christmas at home with my parents and brother the next day.

After spending Christmas at home, everything started to feel real. Right after I came out of my coma, I was afraid to go to sleep at night because I thought this would all turn into another long dream. When I was in a coma, I wanted to wake up because I thought was sleeping the day away, but this dream seemed to go on forever. I would fall asleep early, trying to stay up until 9 p.m. when the hospital turned off the phones for the night, but sometimes I fell asleep before, and then I'd wake up at a bizarre hour at night, like 3 or 4 a.m. and talk to the nurses or just lay there until Mom came at 7 a.m. If she was 2 or 3 minutes past 7, I'd tease her and say that she's late. But after that Christmas break, I could sleep through the night. I knew it was all real then.

Life is real, life is happening. Life goes on, and sometimes we can be very thankful for that life.

C'est la Vie...That's life, and that's how it's gonna be—it just matters what you do with that life. Whether it's your first chance or second, take that opportunity to do something important and worthwhile. Follow your passions because tomorrow is not an absolute guarantee.

My passion for helping others emerged from my accident experience, and I want to help others in similar situations. I know how hard it is to be in the hospital or a rehab center, with nothing fun to do but the free-time activities provided by the staff. So after graduating high school in 2000, when I was 19 years old, I started looking into schools with Therapeutic Recreation programs, which provides activities to people in a hospital, or another inpatient setting. I found Longwood University to have the best program in the state. While visiting the campus, I fell in love with the small size and friendly atmosphere; when I started school in August 2000, I knew I had made the best decision of my life in attending. Close to home, it was still far enough away to where I could feel independent—which is something that I needed at that time in my life. I had just graduated high school and was still in the process of growing up, learning to be on my own, yet I still needed support after just having recovered from a life-changing car accident. The Academic Support Center at

Longwood is wonderful, and was located directly across the street from my dorm building. The staff almost felt like a second family. I would spend many hours there getting help with my classes, or enjoy it as a safe haven in which to come and study.

After graduating Longwood University with a therapeutic recreation degree, I started working in a nursing home assisting residents in the activity department in 2005. I met my husband in 2006; he had looked for similar Longwood alumni on a social networking website, and saw that we had also both attended the same high school, but never met until after college graduation. We bonded over coffee about our love for Longwood. We got married in 2008, adopted a dog, and bought a cute little townhouse.

Danielle is a graduate of Longwood University 2005, earning a bachelor's of science degree in Therapeutic Recreation. She worked in a nursing home for 9 years, and is now spreading TBI awareness through her blog, TBI triumphs. She lives in Northern Virginia with her husband and dog Chazz, is very active in her church, and practices yoga to help her balance both physically and mentally www.tbitriumps.com.

Chapter Twenty-Four
Beyond Survival

Darcy L. Keith
Fishers, Indiana

The stretch of road from Muncie, Indiana, to Morehead, Kentucky, is only 280 miles long—a drive normally lasting less than six hours. When in 1991, I started out on that road as an ambitious college senior, little did I know that my life and dreams for the future would come to a screeching halt in a matter of hours, not to mention that two of my closest friends would be dead.

Everything physically, mentally, emotionally, and financially that I had accomplished in my short life thus far was gone forever. Or was it?

In early September of my senior year, four sorority sisters and I were asked by our national sorority to help start a new chapter at Morehead State University. Currently serving as rush chairman, I happily agreed. But after we completed the rush parties and were returning to Ball State University that evening, something went terribly wrong. As we entered the southern outskirts of Cincinnati, our driver lost control of our vehicle in the wind shear caused by two passing semis. The car spun, and we ended up sideways in the middle of the northbound lanes of the highway, trapped in the path of an approaching semi-tractor trailer. The resulting impact was so great that our car's crumpled side panel bore the imprint of the semi's front license plate.

When the screeching and grinding came to a halt, the two girls buckled in the front seats were able to exit the car and walk away. The three unbuckled girls in the back, including myself, weren't so lucky. Two were killed instantly. The paramedics could not tell at first whether I had survived the crash because they couldn't find my pulse; they had to remove some of my nail polish to be sure. If I were dead, the color under my fingernails would have been blue. It was pink.

Barely breathing and placed on life support, I was rushed by a Life Flight helicopter to the University Of Cincinnati Hospital, and admitted to the surgical critical-care unit.

The injuries I sustained were massive. Unconscious, I remained in a coma for six days with a frontal lobe and left-brain injuries that paralyzed my body's right side. The doctors told my parents that the prognosis was grim. Damage to the left side of my brain resulted in a significant loss of memory, and also impaired my motor skills. Brain bruising, bleeding, and swelling in my frontal lobe caused brain cells to die, which left a gaping hole. Damage was done, but the extent was still unknown.

Awaking from my coma, I was scared and confused. With no control over my bodily functions, I endured the humiliation of adult diapers. Due to the right extremity paralysis, getting around required the use of a wheelchair. Also paralyzed was my right vocal cord, which initially left me unable to speak. My right lung collapsed, and I also experienced foot drop. Eating was very difficult as well, since I was unable to swallow. A feeding tube that went up my nose and down my throat to my stomach nourished me daily. When I was finally able to feed myself, I was put in a special feeding group to learn how to swallow again. Once I mastered the swallowing process, I graduated to eating "normal" everyday food items.

It was during a session with all my therapists present that I learned of the car crash and the deaths of my two sorority sisters. As I sat in shock and disbelief upon hearing the news, the therapists watched closely to see my reaction. I could only utter the words, "Why didn't I die?" No one replied except my mother, but to this day, I can't recall what she said to me. I couldn't believe that they were dead, but the scars on my body told me that something terrible had happened.

At first, my only thought was about how to survive my injuries. Beside my hospital bed was a chart listing various tasks that I would have to complete independently before I could be discharged. I refused to dwell on my injuries or give up hope. Completing each task became my new goal. With determination, I began relearning simple skills like brushing my teeth, dressing myself, tying my shoes, and going to the bathroom. I progressed to more complex skills like eating, walking, and behaving normally for someone my age. Occupational and speech therapy helped get my brain back on track cognitively. During physical therapy, when placed upright, I was like a bobble head doll from lack of neck and trunk support. When I started getting some feeling back from the paralysis, the pain was so intense that I whimpered continuously. This feeling was like pins and needles constantly poking me in my arm and leg. But despite the excruciating pain, I learned how to stand and walk without falling over from my balance issues. Slowly, one by one, each item on my bedside chart was completed and checked off.

Emotionally though, I was still struggling. Having a brain injury is similar to having attention deficit disorder (ADD). I didn't have the attention span to focus on the information I wanted to remember. I couldn't concentrate enough to remember it, or recall what I just did. Damage to my brain's left lobe left me with memory loss of my entire college major. When one of my college textbooks was placed on the table in front of me at the hospital, I just looked at it in a blank stare. No longer could I perform the required math tasks needed for my actuarial-science college major. In fact, I couldn't remember anything related to the subject.

Before the crash, I was going to be walking onstage draped in a bright red cap and gown, ready to receive my diploma. Now, with college graduation just six months away, this was no longer an option for me.

How was I going to provide for myself financially if I couldn't graduate from college and get a job? My self-esteem and self-confidence plummeted. *It took all the strength I had not to fall apart.*

Extremely upset and emotional, I searched for what options were available for my "new normal" status. Not only would I learn how to survive—I would thrive. I had all my life to live, and I was not about to throw it away after being given a second chance. I wasn't about to feel sorry for myself. Developing a memorable recipe for overcoming adversity and dealing with change, I began on a mission to rebuild my life. Working out consisted of brisk, long walks and light strength training. To mend and re-engage my brain, I re-enrolled in college under a new major, and graduated a short year and a half later, as determined as ever. The company with whom I had interned offered me a job in a different capacity.

Holding my head up high, I continued to grow and flourish with determination and a positive attitude. To turn a devastating situation into a positive one, I went on a mission to help others live better lives by sharing my formula of overcoming adversity and making good decisions. I did this by serving as a professional keynote speaker for various organizations, associations, and corporations.

As college students, we make some pretty poor choices. Had the three of us in the back seat thought about the consequences of not wearing our seat belts, my friends would still be with us, and I wouldn't have sustained my life-altering injuries. Instead, I made a conscious effort to not wear one. The reason? I didn't want to wrinkle my clothes, since I was going to a party when returning to college. Pretty lame decision, isn't it? That choice nearly cost me my life, and unfortunately, my friends paid the ultimate price.

By retelling the story and the vital lessons learned from this tragedy, I have been blessed with the opportunity to not only help countless individuals and organizations overcome adversity and successfully deal with change, but also keep my friends' memories alive. Several NFL teams have invited me to annually present the "Traffic Education and Decision Making" module of the NFL Rookie Success Program to their new rookie class. My story and subsequent consequences of making a poor decision are "incredibly powerful" to the rookies, as I was their age when I made that tragic and life-altering choice.

I choose to live each day to the fullest. I don't dwell on things I can't control, nor do I take a "victim" attitude. Despite the obstacles ahead, I choose to embrace them with perseverance and fortitude. I don't allow my ego to get the best of me, but ask for help when it was needed. All of these elements helped me become the professional speaker, author, leader, and advocate that I am today.

The stretch of road from Muncie, Indiana, to Morehead, Kentucky, is only 280 miles long—a drive normally lasting less than six hours. But while everything did come to a screeching halt for a time, my life was far from being over. In fact, it had just begun.

Darcy L. Keith is a national award-winning Professional Inspirational Speaker and a survivor of two traumatic brain injuries. Serving on the advisory committee of the Ohio Valley Center for Brain Injury Prevention and Rehabilitation at Ohio State University since 1999, and on the Brain Board of Directors for the Brain Injury Association of Indiana from 2003-12, she is a contributing author to five books of various topics. Darcy has appeared on various television and radio venues and serves as a keynote speaker on the topic of brain injury and overcoming adversity for various conferences, corporations, non-profits, associations, colleges, and for the National Football League (NFL) Rookie Success Program. www.DarcyKeith.com

Chapter Twenty-Five
Adopting a Never-Give-Up Attitude

David Rowlands
Sydney, Australia

On a hot sunny afternoon in March 2009 in Brisbane, Australia, I was riding my bicycle home from my job at a local military facility. I was wearing an approved bicycle helmet and high visibility clothing. I had been working in the job for around six months.

I was very fit for a 60-year-old. About a mile from home as I was travelling through an intersection at about 25 mph, and in my peripheral vision, I saw the flash of a vehicle approaching from behind and then turn across my path. There was not enough time to brake, and as I screamed out at the driver, the front of my bicycle went under the front wheel of the vehicle. Momentum propelled me over the front, and I remember being spun end-over-end in midair.

When I regained consciousness, I was strapped to an ambulance litter and had on a neck brace. I was told later that I had been lying on the road for some time, and that two doctors from a nearby medical center who had been passing by had stabilized me before the ambulance arrived. In the ER, I was examined for skull, spinal and neck injuries, and due to the abrasions on my right shoulder, there was concern that it was fractured. I had sustained a 2" crack in the back of my skull and bruising to the right temporal lobe. I felt no pain due to the morphine, and I thought that I was lucid and making sense. I expected that I would be released and allowed to go home to my wife and family. That was not to be so.

I spent the next three days flat on my back with the neck brace on, and pleaded with the hospital staff to have it removed due to the discomfort. After the neck brace was removed, I sat up and the room started spinning uncontrollably. Any slight head movement gave me severe vertigo. I fought through it because I wanted so much to get out of the hospital. I staggered up and down the hallway like a drunk, forcing myself upright for the next five days. The morphine had worn off and the pain was surprisingly intense. My body hurt all over, and my brain was in a fog-like state. My daughter told me later that I was not making sense when she visited me in hospital.

After the eight days in hospital I was discharged and went home. I had no idea how damaged my body was until I decided to take a walk to the local shopping center. It was a trip I had done many times before, and I used to power walk there and back. The reality hit me hard on the way home because I had to stop many times to rest by sitting down wherever I could. I was stunned at how weak I had become.

A week later I was receiving physiotherapy for my injured shoulder, and was given exercises to do with elastic bands to build up strength in the supporting shoulder muscles. A month after my hospital discharge, I attended a review by the treating neurosurgeon. He had the CT scan images of my skull on his laptop, and in the process of viewing it, was surprised to find that I also had damage to my left middle ear. He told me then I was kept in the hospital for so long because they anticipated I would have seizures due to my brain injury.

It was expected that I would return to work through a workcover insurance program where I would have a gradual increase in hours and days. I had to be examined by a specialist engaged by the insurance company, and he deemed that I had severe positional vertigo, and referred me to a colleague who specialized in that field. He really wanted me to see an equilibrium physiotherapist. When it was determined that I had three separate types of vertigo, I underwent testing and was assigned a set of exercises as therapy.

I was determined to overcome the vertigo because my life was on hold until then. There was improvement in the range of movement in my shoulder, and the torn muscles in my abdomen and contusions in other areas had stopped hurting.

My recovery took seven months before I was able to drive and work full time. But I faced another obstacle. My job was physically demanding and after a full week of work, I was totally spent. I slept most of the weekend trying to build up my strength to face another week. I was fighting a losing battle. Despite my best efforts, I was forced to resign from my job in July 2010. It was then that I started to unravel. I suffered severe depression and had thoughts of suicide. My life had fallen apart, and then my wife abandoned me, taking our pre-teen son and the family car. I was left to clean up the mess and sell the family home. I was fortunate that I had help from my wife's family, and the house was sold quickly.

I am financially settled now, and I moved to my home city of Sydney about two years ago to live with a woman I had known in my teenage years. Things went very well for a while, but then she realized I was damaged goods, and forced me to move out of her home. I live in a share house now and I am happy. I write and perform songs and have a regular dance partner who tells me that I am "the best dance partner ever." I am blessed to have friends and family who understand and do not judge me, and accept me the way I am. There is hope that I may regain more cognitive power.

My biggest obstacles are: short-term memory loss, lack of focus, loss of drive to get things done, disrupted sleep patterns, chronic fatigue, anxiety, PTSD, and loss of libido. I have learned to manage these challenges.

I want others who read my story to know that there is hope and the opportunity for things to improve over time. Remaining positive has been my most powerful tool. I came out of severe depression a survivor—and learned strategies to stop that from ever happening again.

My message to the world is that no matter how bad things may seem, the future holds hope for us all.

I would like my story to inspire others to adopt a positive, never-give-up attitude to their situation, and to count every day as a blessing. Seize the moment and celebrate the joy of life with your family and friends. Most of all, be good to yourself.

David acquired a TBI from a motor vehicle turning across his path in 2009. He was thrown from his bicycle, landing head first on the road. He sustained a fractured skull and bruising to his right temporal lobe. His recovery has been a long process, and he is seeing improvements in his condition.

Chapter Twenty-Six
I Will Fly With Broken Wings

Deep (last name withheld)
Mumbai, India

I was working with one of the best companies in India. I was recently married, and was happy because both my professional and personal life was excellent. My wife and I had dreams, goals, and aspirations to achieve at this, the start of our new life. My wife was getting used to fast-paced Mumbai life where she moved post-marriage, and was searching for a job.

I was flying high until…it is well said that you never know what the next moment holds for you.

We left our home at 4 p.m. September 5, 2015. We did not know at that moment we were never going to return to our home that we had made with love. This was our dream home, even though it was rented apartment, because there resides our love, our dreams, our smiles, and each and every moment of happiness and giggles.

Driving along, there was a BANG! The young driver crashed into us, which changed our lives forever. I am no longer the person I was, and have no answer whether I will ever be what I was.

After the accident, both of us are in the ICU. My and my wife's parents are waiting outside ICU, wondering: will our son make it; will our son-in-law make it, will he be alive or be able to walk again. When my sister is notified, she takes the first flight to India from USA. I wonder what was going on in her mind: Will I be able to see my brother alive, or will I lose him forever even before I reach him?

My wife had a severe leg injury, which itself was very critical because she could not walk for next six months, but she also had concussion, and first two days, September 9 and 10, were deleted from her memory, and she still doesn't remember it after coming back to her senses. My poor girl was in pain, but she could not feel her pain as she watched her husband lying in bed in front of her in a coma.

I was in coma for 12 days—this is what I'm told as I don't remember it. These 12 days doctors had no answer to my loved ones' questions, and although he could see the pain fear in their eyes, even he was helpless. Even though the science of medicine has progressed, only God has certain answers. Once I came out of the coma, my loved ones had more concerns about what my life would be now as I suffered a traumatic brain injury. I had lost my memory, cognitive skills, could not walk or talk, and for that matter, did not even know the difference between day and night.

I did fight hard to come out of the coma, but my real life battle would start now, relearning everything.

When I was conscious, I did not recognize my loving sweetheart wife, but I did recognize my mom. Now I understand why they say you remember your mother when you are in pain as she has carried you in her womb for nine months. I had lost a part of my life, and remember only my early years, so I remembered people who were part of my childhood.

And here I am back to life after being in a state of unconscious, but my real struggle starts now on this journey with traumatic brain injury. I have a new life where I am reborn and where I will have to relearn to eat, walk, talk, read, and write. An MBA who has worked with the best companies, I now have to start again with the A-B-Cs. What a life.

Welcome to my 15-month journey, which will take you through pain, fear, baby steps to moving ahead, emotions, love, care, and the end may be take you closer to understanding true love.

After 21 days in hospital, I was back home physically—but I am no longer the same as I was 21 days ago. That Deep is lost, he is dead, and it's a new person who is here. Yes, I was back home in 21 days—because we don't have rehabilitation centers or any rehabilitation program which could at least help me relearn to do basic things like to brush my teeth, comb my hair and shave. Now I returned home, and my mom took me back like I a newborn. She is a strong woman who took up the challenge to make me stand up on my legs within one month. Of course the doctors thought she is being emotional, that standing was not possible. Completing hospital formalities to leave took a whole day. My first night at home was a nightmare, and most difficult one for my mom because I messed my pants three times. I wonder how she managed to clean me, but she did because that's what a mother is all about. This was the start to long, painful journey.

As the days passed, I start doing basic things on my own after first being guided by my mom. Without any rehabilitation centers or programs, it was all up to my family members and my will to relearn. My right side was not functioning at all, my right hand was fractured, but my legs were fine except the connection between my legs and brain was a problem. If I were instructed to pick up my left leg and walk, it would not do that, so to address this, a physiotherapist did come three days a week for three months. I walked and used my right hand perfectly, which was some relief to my loved ones.

My favorite aunt is a schoolteacher who taught me to talk again as I used to speak with a lisp, and sometimes I was inarticulate. She was my speech therapist for a month, coming every morning and going to her home late evening, so whenever I was not sleeping, she was talking to me. For a few months, I did sleep alot, and that's why my brain healed faster. My mom made sure she gave me good nutrition for my brain health, but it meant spending lot of her time in the kitchen and cooking it herself because we Indians believe homemade food is best for health. Yes, it did prove very beneficial to me. My home is my rehabilitation center, with a physiotherapist, speech therapist, nutritionist and everyone all giving their best.

But the most important person in my life is missing—I might not remember her because of my memory loss—but my heart was surely missing her and was in pain because my brain had lost the connection, but we were still connected by our hearts. This was the worst part of my journey as my wife had suffered leg injury, and because we could no longer pay rent, I was staying at my parents' place and she was staying at relatives' homes because my parents' home was small and could not accommodate her.

So days and weeks passed, and my mom was doing her best to make me stand and walk. With her and the physiotherapist's efforts, I was walking without any support within month, and when I walked to my psychiatrist, he was quite shocked, but after a few seconds, he stood up from his chair and hugged me. He thought I would not walk, at least not so soon. He, my neurologist and other doctors thought I would be in a vegetative state. So now I walked to him and talked to him because my aunt's speech therapy had done miracles for me. From here started my one-hour sessions with a psychiatrist. He remarked that I was talking sense, but my memory was a concern because I forgot what I had talked about a few minutes ago, and would lose the link between conversations. According to him, my intellectuals were perfect; the affected area of the brain was the emotional part. He was right as even today I get angry about small things, and sometimes I get so emotional that I cry.

I think nobody can ever understand the pain my wife was going through. She had a concussion and leg injury, and was on complete bed rest, but the worst pain was being separated from her husband. Because she could not walk, she could come to meet me. Because I did not remember her, I did not call her. But my aunt and my friends who came to visit me made sure I talked to her, even if it was for only few seconds. When I did, most surprisingly, I talked to her in same way that I used to, telling her, "I love you, I miss you," but after some time, I would forget she is my wife. She was lonely, she was in pain, she needed her husband, and her husband doesn't even remember her.

As time passed, I was healing and so was she. Physically, I had drastically improved, and I was getting my memory back. I initially remembered her as my girlfriend as we talked over phone. She was one who was reading and researching about traumatic brain injury, and my sister was doing same thing from USA, so both suggested that cognitive rehabilitation is what needs to be started. The next step would be relearning to read and write. Although my wife was not with me, on phone she instructed me to write the ABCs in a book.

Yes, I had to start with ABCs. As a professor she wanted to teach me best, and made sure I wrote and sent her picture on the phone so she could check. Then ABC got converted into paragraphs. She made me write things I saw in books; then she dictated to me on phone. When I wrote and sent her pictures, she then gave grade marks. It sounds funny, but that's what made us walk through it.

Then three months later, she left her relatives' place and came to my parents' home. We started living together, but this was start of other tough times as there was not a room in this house for us, so we had to sleep in the hall. It is indeed the worst situation in my life where I have to make my wife sleep in a hall where we have no privacy. Once she was back, she brought in books for cognitive skills and started training me; then she had me work on a laptop, and eventually trained me on the professional work I did at my job. I am lucky that my employer is indeed one of the best because they not only waited for me, but I went back to the same position I had before. I have started going to the office, but I have my set of challenges like memory problem, problem in cognitive skills, and aphasia. My wife and I have designed strategies to deal with it, like for memory, I write down each thing I do at the office. My boss and colleagues are also very helpful.

I would like to tell all the survivors to keep fighting, and you will get through it. Yes, of course, we are not the same as we were and can never be, but once you accept it, you will find ways to move forward. Love yourself. And to all caregivers, thank you for being with us as we could not walk this path without you.

In this journey of mine, those who have contributed include my parents, my sister, my doctors and my wife. I will be always thankful and obliged to them because without them I could not have been on the path of recovery.

I feel pain for my wife because she has compromised and given up everything for me, and is standing strong by me even when she knows our future is uncertain. We don't know how our future life will be with my TBI, but she is and will be with me.

My wings are broken but my desire and determination to fly are still alive, and I will fly with my broken wings. I want to fly because I see unconditional love in eyes of my wife—*and for her I have to.*

No bio provided, and written anonymously for personal reasons

Chapter Twenty-Seven
The Magic of Music

Derek A. O'Neal
Alexandria, Virginia

Please keep in mind that this is not a research-based presentation. This is simply my story…my life, my accident, the role music played in my recovery, and my ongoing journey as a brain injury survivor.

Early on, in my work together with my good friend, the late Christine Schneider of Hope Rehabilitation Network in East Lansing, Michigan, I was told that I possessed a passion for a number of things, not the least of which was music. So, right from the start, music became and continues to play a major role and is always an important part of our discussions.

•••••

Welcome to our presentation, The Magic of Music! I am extremely honored to be here with you today, and to have this opportunity to speak about my journey as a brain injury survivor.

To give you a little background: I grew up in New York City and am the oldest of nine children. I attended Stuyvesant High School, the College Of William & Mary, Embry-Riddle Aeronautical University, and the United States Army Command & General Staff College. I have a Bachelor of Science Degree in Professional Aeronautics, and a Master of Science Degree in Military Science. I retired from the United States Army in 1996 and am very proud of my career. A few of the highlights of my military career include my designation as the Army's Air Traffic Controller of the Year in 1984m and command of an Armored Cavalry Unit in 1991 during Operations Desert Shield and Desert Storm while serving in Iraq and Kuwait. When I joined the Army in 1981 was when I served as an Air Traffic Controller.

When the Army discovered that I had already had a college education, they recommended that I attempt to qualify for the Army Officer Candidate School (OCS). I was accepted to attend OCS and received an Officer Commission in 1985 as a Lieutenant. In 1989, I was promoted to Captain while stationed in what was then the Federal Republic of Germany. I lived in Mainz and served as an Air Defense Artillery Officer.

Additionally, in 1989, I was transferred back to United States to the Army Armor Branch where I became an Armored Cavalry Officer. I was assigned to the Third Armored Cavalry Regiment at Fort Bliss in El Paso, Texas (3 ACR). I proudly served my nation and was willing participant of the Gulf War. Upon conclusion of the war, I was selected to become a member of the Army Inspector General (IG) Corps, but I decided I would take advantage of the United States Military post-Gulf War Draw Down plan and accept retirement in 1996. I was promoted to Major and was eager to retire and move on with my life.

I am married to my high school sweetheart, Rene', and together we have five children—three in college, one in high school, and one in elementary school.

My brain injury occurred on June 7, 2004 while driving home from work. I was traveling on the freeway at approximately 70 mph when suddenly a deer ran in front of my car. The deer smashed through my windshield, and was killed instantly. However, the impact of the collision caused my vehicle to crash.

When I was found, I was transported to a level-one trauma center, William Beaumont Hospital in Royal Oak, Michigan. While at Beaumont, I required two brain surgeries, and remained in a coma for almost month. About seven weeks after my accident, I was transferred to Hope Network where my intensive rehabilitation began.

Now, you remember that I am a former military officer. Well, early in my recovery, I actually believed that I was a Prisoner Of War (POW).

I actually remember trying to escape from Hope Network whenever the opportunity presented itself. I remember asking my young son to unlock doors for me, realizing that at three years old, he had no idea what I was planning. I remember Dr. Cooke addressing me in a military manner by calling me Major O'Neal, and I remember that when he addressed me in that fashion, I would respond immediately because I remembered that in the Army, all doctors were commissioned military officers, and in many cases held a higher military rank than their patients.

So much for my military memories. Now it's time to discuss much more pleasant issues.

I also love to sing, and for some reason, the Hope Network contingent tolerated my singing and encouraged me to sing often. It is very true that music did many things for me, and most importantly, what it did for me initially was help me remember. While I was struggling to make sense of who I was, music seemed to tap into my memories. I'd listen to a tune and rhythm of a song, and soon find myself singing some words. And the more I sang, the more words I'd remember. One of my early favorites was "Loving You" by Minnie Ripperton. I remember that I believed the words were so appropriate to dedicate to my lovely wife Rene.'

Interestingly enough, I remember asking one of the Hope Network therapists an important question: Who was the beautiful woman who visits me often? When I was told that she was my wife, I was ecstatic! I said to myself, if this Derek O'Neal guy is married to this gorgeous woman, he must have been okay!

Whenever I think of what she went through while she assisted with my recovery, I'm reminded *what the real definition of love is.*

The words of "Loving You" are so appropriate and the lyrics are a love song… "Loving you is easy because you're beautiful."

(In my presentations, I sing the whole song, but for this story, I'll simply give you the song's strong message.)

So, the people at Hope Network signed me up to attend music therapy at Michigan State University once a week.

"According to the American Music Therapy Association, "the idea of music as a healing influence which could affect health and behavior is at least as old as the writings of Aristotle and Plato. The 20th Century discipline began after World War I and World War II when community musicians of all types, both amateur and professional, went to Veteran's Hospitals around the country to play for thousands of Veteran's suffering from both physical and emotional trauma from the wars."

"The patients' notable physical and emotional responses to music led the doctors and nurses to request the hiring of musicians by the hospitals. It was soon evident that hospital musicians needed some prior training before entering the facility so demand grew for a college curriculum. The first Music Therapy degree program in the world, founded at Michigan State University in 1944, celebrated its 50th Anniversary in 1994. The American Music Therapy Association was founded in 1998...."

So how does music affect us? Music promotes:

- vocalization
- rhythmic movements
- orientation
- relaxation
- self-expression
- self esteem

Where do we find music? Where did it begin? There is and always will be music in every culture. It's an integral part of our most important human events: birth, death, love, political and social expression, war. and religion. No one knows exactly when music began. Our ancestors may have tapped something out on stones or wood.

Yes, music did help me. I love all music but I guess that jazz and Motown tunes are my favorite. So, for days and evenings, I filled the hallways of Hope Network with my favorite tunes. I found that the music did two things for me: 1) It energized me, and 2) It made and kept me very happy.

I loved singing so much that, even on outings to the mall, I would sing. My teenaged children, however, gave me some immediate feedback on that. I quickly learned that while singing at Hope Network was acceptable, singing at the mall with teenagers *was absolutely not*.

What I really want to share about the affect that music had on me during the early stages of my recovery is this: for me, *music was healing*. Music stirred my emotions and feelings, and enabled me to deal with my grief, sadness, and anger. And there always seemed to be a song that fit.

When I was sad, there was "Don't Worry Be Happy" by Bobby McFerrin. His song tells us that in every life we have some troubles, but don't worry, be happy.

When I awoke and started my day, there was "Lovely Day" by Bill Withers. His song says that on those difficult and challenging days, I look at you, my love, and it *is a lovely day*.

It always made me feel very good when people responded positively to my songs. I enjoyed seeing their smiles. It felt even better when some would join in with me, and maybe even get up to dance and/or clap their hands.

So, what is my take-away message?

Remember that music touches the soul, nourishes us, and has the power to soothe, inspire, invigorate, and keep you well. So, for all of us who have been affected by brain injury—whether you are a victim, family member, or friend—there is an appropriate song that I want to leave you with today, titled "Life Is A Song Worth Singing." This song's message is that you are strong and not helpless. You can decide what to do with your life. You contain the power in your mind to control your destiny.

Derek is married to his high school sweetheart, Rene' Stewart O'Neal. He is the father of five children. Four are college graduates and one attends high school. His education includes the College of William and Mary and Embry-Riddle Aeronautical University. He is a retired United States Army Officer who is an Operation Desert Storm veteran. In June of 2004, he suffered a Brain Injury when his car hit a deer while he was driving home. After his recovery, he pursued and received a Post-Graduate credential as a Paralegal and began this new phase of his career. He was a Paralegal Specialist at the United States Department of Justice in Washington, DC. Antitrust Division. Prior to his car/deer accident in 2004, he managed many manufacturing assembly companies while rising to the position of Vice President of Operations at an Automotive Assembly Holding Group I Michigan. Additionally, he was a Board Member of the Brain Injury Association of Michigan for six years and is now a Board Member of the Brain Injury Association of Virginia.

Chapter Twenty-Eight
The Day That Changed Everything

Diane Keyes
Minneapolis, Minnesota

Everything changed for me one beautiful August morning in 1955, the month before I was to start fourth grade. It's easy to pinpoint the exact time because I had a brain hemorrhage that day. I was sitting on the sofa watching "Axel and His Dog," a popular local children's TV show, and eating red licorice. Then I got a blinding headache.

Mom was downstairs doing laundry so I staggered across what instantly seemed like a much larger living room to the basement door, bouncing off the sofa, end table and hallway wall as I went. I had barely enough time to call down to her before my legs buckled beneath me. In the few seconds it took Mom to reach me, I passed out, and she scrambled to the phone for help.

I could hear her screaming out the back door to our next-door neighbors, "Ralph, Florence, come quick, help me, something has happened to Diane." They laid me gently on the bed and waited for what must have seemed like an eternity until the ambulance came. I remember trying to say something to reassure Mom, but I couldn't move a muscle or open my eyes.

I don't recall anything more until I "woke up" to find myself looking down on me—the physical me—lying on an operating table, surrounded by several doctors working to save my life. Although it sounds like it must have been very scary, I had no sense of anxiety or fear, just the comforting knowledge that my body was entirely separate from the "real" me. Even now, I can instantly bring to mind, with great clarity, the profound sense of well-being I experienced during the time I spent in both worlds. That memory has been a comfort to me my entire life.

As I hovered near the ceiling, I could see Mom frantically waiting in another room for news of my condition. I wanted to comfort her, tell her, "Mom, don't worry, I'm just fine," but, instinctively, I knew I was simply an observer and unable to participate in what was happening.

You may think that what happened to me took place in my imagination, in an anesthetically induced dream state. I wondered too. But God soon gave me proof I hadn't imagined what I remember so vividly.

While I was floating blissfully in the in-between space above my body, I noticed one of the physicians assisting with the surgery. Her sure hands and deft movements mesmerized me. In the 1950s, a woman doctor was rare. A Korean woman doctor working in a hospital in St. Paul, Minnesota was as rare as, say—an out-of-body-experience. Small and soft-spoken, with a slight limp and a broad smile, I instantly recognized her when she came into my room to visit me a few days later. I hadn't dreamed what happened, it was real!

I went to Catholic school and attended Mass every morning. Like my classmates, by the tender age of eight, I'd memorized much of the Baltimore Catechism—the primer of my Catholic faith doctrine. But my faith had been just a word. Defined in the dictionary, faith means "belief without proof." Now I had proof. My out-of-body experience gave me proof—personal knowledge about the eternal me.

So many meant-to-be moments came together that day to save and change my life. Our doctor, Dr. A., was Dad's bowling buddy, a member of our church, and the doctor who delivered me. He lived only a few blocks away from our home in Roseville, and arrived at the hospital even before the ambulance. A man of deep faith, he went to Mass every morning.

His faith touched every aspect of his life, and on that particular day it touched mine as well. As he raced to the emergency room, something told him I needed a spinal tap. As soon as I arrived, he performed the procedure, right then and there. That must have been the point when, close to death, the real "me" awakened to usher my eternal self to glory. I'm not sure what brought me back—most likely, it was the sight of Mom, and the anguish she so obviously felt at the thought of losing me.

Many years later, at Dad's funeral, Dr. A. told me he felt guided by the Holy Spirit to do a spinal tap on me that day. I have no doubt that is true. Nothing but divine guidance could compel most physicians to take such extreme measures in the absence of any concrete evidence.

Probably because of the extraordinary experience I had at such a young age, I deeply believe in the power of prayer to change our hearts and bring the word of God close enough for us to hear it. So it doesn't surprise me that someone who took time from his hectic schedule each day to spend time in prayer and meditation would have access to Divine inspiration.

The incredibly brave and rash decision Dr. A. made to follow his own meant-to-be guidance, relieved the pressure in my brain and saved my life that morning so many years ago. When I think of the risk he took for me, I am filled with profound gratitude for the value he placed on my life, and awe at his dedication to his vocation and his willingness to follow the promptings of the Spirit.

I was given a great gift that day. Since the moment I looked down on myself in the ER, I have had no fear of death—that fear left me the moment I knew that my body was not me but only a shell that contained my spirit as long as I needed it. I've learned since that an event such as this is called a "touchstone moment" because it remains in your heart—always ready to comfort and sustain you whenever it's needed. And it has.

But I received an even greater gift as well. What happened made me feel that my very survival was meant-to-be. I overheard enough people whispering in the corridor outside my room to know that most people who had brain hemorrhages died. Today, brain hemorrhages are fatal for more than 25 percent of people suffering them. In the 1950s, they killed nine out of ten victims. Lying in my hospital bed, I had a lot of time to think about my near-death experience and that I was still alive.

Why had God spared my life? Living with that question changed me. At age eight, I was already on a spiritual quest—one that has lasted the rest of my life. My longing to find an answer has led me down roads I might never have chosen without it. I worked in parish ministry for many years, accompanied my husband through his training to become a deacon, earning the equivalent of a master's degree in theology, and taking another 3 year course to become a spiritual counselor.

Over the years, I've asked myself countless times: Is this it? Is this the reason I was spared? While I've never felt with certainty that my search was over—I've learned, as Rainer Maria Rilke said, to "Be patient toward all that is unsolved…and try to love the questions themselves…. Live the questions now." And although I still haven't found an answer, my quest has lead me down interesting roads and I wouldn't change a thing.

Diane has been a home stager for more than 30 years and a spiritual director since 1999. An award-winning author, Diane Keyes' children's book, "Spirit of the Snowpeople," sold out its first printing in three weeks. Her home-staging book, "This Sold House," is soon to be in its fourth printing and her memoir, "To Wendy's With Love: The Twenty-Two Year Lunch," will be released in November 2016.

Chapter Twenty-Nine
Nightmare in the TBI Disability Lane

Donna O'Donnell Figurski
Surprise, Arizona

I'm living a nightmare, and I'm glad that I am. Sounds strange, huh. Who would want to be trapped in a nightmare every waking moment? Well, I don't want to be trapped here, but here I am nonetheless. I would prefer to take back my happy, secure life with my husband, David…taking long walks each evening, going out on weekends for date nights, and strolling through the parks on Sunday mornings to our favorite breakfast restaurant.

But, on January 13, 2005, when David was 57-years-old our lives burst when something burst inside his head. The doctors call it a TBI, a traumatic brain injury. *I call it a living nightmare.*

My nightmare began when David's head filled with blood from exercising too much. He was in excruciating pain. He was moaning and writhing on the bed, sweat pouring from his body. When the paramedics finally placed the oxygen mask over David's face, relief came—for David and for me. He became silent, and I was grateful. He looked peaceful, but I soon realized that he had slipped into a coma. My calm was an illusion because a coma was not good.

When David arrived at the emergency room, the doctor sent him for a CAT scan of his brain, and decided to perform immediate surgery to evacuate the blood from the massive hematoma. When I met the neurosurgeon, he said that he'd examined David's brain on his home computer, and came in immediately. His words boosted me. "Your husband is in good shape." But his next words plunged me into despair. "He will make a great organ donor." His pronouncement left me in shock. But, there were more surprises. After David's surgery, which he wasn't expected to survive, his neurosurgeon relayed the results of the surgery. He proudly told me he had saved David's life. I was elated. But again, his next words floored me. "Your husband is a professor. He won't want to be a vegetable. If he doesn't improve by morning, we'll pull the plug." I clenched my hands and was silent, but my mind whirred. I had to get David to his home hospital of Columbia Presbyterian in New York City, where he was a professor in the Department of Microbiology.

Against the advice of the neurosurgeon at this first hospital, David was transferred to Columbia Presbyterian Hospital where his new doctor found an aneurysm, which needed to be removed immediately. During that second surgery, an arterial venous malformation (AVM) was discovered, which also needed to be excised. David had three emergency brain surgeries in less than two weeks.

For each surgery, David had a slight chance to live. Still, I had to sign on the dotted line. David's life was in my hands. I wanted to ask him if he wanted this surgery. We always conferred on important decisions, and this was the most important one of our lives. I wanted to shake him awake. I needed to know if I was making the right decision, but he lay "sleeping" in his coma. He remained that way for several weeks, and I had to make the hardest decisions of my life—alone. And so I signed again and again. I had no choice. If the operations were not performed, David would surely die, and I could not live without him.

Although David is a survivor, having battled three brain surgeries, the nightmare continues. The brain trauma affected his motor skills and had reduced his mobility to almost an infantile stage. He had to relearn to walk. His balance was, and is still, greatly affected. Although he has made significant gains, he has a long road to travel.

For the first month after the surgeries, David remained in the Neurological Intensive Care Unit (NICU) and then the step-down unit in preparation for discharge. While there, the right side of his body was near-paralyzed. Within four weeks, as David became more aware, he slowly regained movement. Then he moved to a rehabilitation hospital, where he began the struggle to relearn to walk. At that time, the best way to describe David was that he was "like a rag doll." He had as much balance and coordination as Raggedy

Andy. Even when using a walker, David could topple over in a slight breeze.

When, nearly a year later, David began to use a four-pronged cane, he was still shaky and needed to be shadowed everywhere. He was rarely far from my side. David continues to gain strength even now. Progress is steadily being made, though it is taking a very long time. Rebuilding his life will be a lifelong project. Now, David is able to walk on his own, but picture C3PO of "Star Wars" movie. David's walk is very robot-like. He is unsteady and can easily lose his balance, so he still needs someone to be with him in the outside world. But, he is able to maneuver by himself inside our home. That's not to say that I don't worry every waking moment about an unexpected fall, which would set him back.

David's speech was also greatly affected. It was nearly impossible to understand him after they removed the trach. His voice was raspy, and his words were garbled. Fortunately, today, although his voice is still gravelly and his speech is still very pronounced, he can be understood, but he may never regain the same beautiful voice he had before the TBI. Sometimes, I call him "marshmallow-mouth" because it seems as if his words are climbing over marshmallows to get out. That only happens when he is really tired or when he is actually eating marshmallows. "It's hard work to talk," he tells me. I know because I see his silent struggle.

It's natural that most folks take life for granted. It's not until you lose something that you realize how valuable it is. It's not until you have to struggle to attain something that its meaning is redefined.

Eating has become a huge challenge. David prefers soft foods. Chewing is difficult, and he often bites his lip, inner cheek, or tongue when he's eating because of loss of feeling on the right side of his face. While most folks never give a thought to eating, the procedure of stabbing food on a fork, delivering it to one's mouth, chewing, and swallowing has become a deliberate process for David. Another major concern is aspiration where he might inhale food or liquid, which can cause serious medical problems. So, my way of preparing foods has changed drastically to accommodate him. The crockpot has become my best friend because it cooks food to a very soft consistency.

It's also hard work to open a door or brush your teeth when your hand won't cooperate because it shakes uncontrollably with ataxia. It's hard work to stand up or sit down or take a step when you have little balance. It's hard work to take a sip of water, eat a bowl of ice cream, or even sleep when you can't swallow properly, and fear aspiration or choking to death. It's hard work to see double, blurry, and tilted images 24/7. (Well maybe 17/7. I don't think David dreams in double, blurry, and tilted images.) It's hard work to read a computer screen with the font raised to 24 and with the images bouncing around the screen. It's hard work even going to the bathroom—judging from the time it takes—since it takes so long to get there (balance) and unfasten the belt (ataxia). Throw in a little neurogenic bladder disorder and partial paralysis, and it makes for a lot of uncertainty. Living with traumatic brain injury is simply HARD WORK!

It's not easy for David. It's not easy for me either, but we are a team. We have been since we met when I was sixteen and he was seventeen, and knew I would marry him.

David also struggles to overcome the ataxia in his right hand. Shortly after he was released from rehab, he visited my first-grade class. It was an opportunity to raise awareness about brain injury and to make young minds sensitive to people with disabilities. The "kiddles" were vastly curious and excited to meet David. When he visited, he shook hands with each of them. They laughed, all in good humor, while he tried to steady his hand enough to grasp each of theirs.

Fortunately, David has a great attitude; he rarely lets anything get him down. A good outlook is essential because there is no easy, fast way out of this nightmare.

About six months after David's brain injury, while he was at home recuperating, a professor friend asked him to be the keynote speaker at a scientific symposium in Colorado. Though David immediately agreed, I was skeptical. David's speech was still garbled. He was still like a rag doll. But our friend assured me that David could do it, and he wanted no one else. He was right! A year and a half after his brain injury, David presented an hour-long lecture about his work on Aggregatibacter actinomycetemcomitans. (Don't ask me because I haven't a clue. I can't even pronounce it. I just call it by its short name: "AA.") David's talk was well received, and he enjoyed many compliments, not only on the results of his work and that of his students, but also many of the scientists made a point to tell him that he was completely understandable.

It was then, with confidence "in his back pocket," that David began to make arrangements to return to his laboratory at Columbia University. No one thought that David would ever unlock his lab door again, especially Human Resources. Though David's cognitive brain was entirely intact, his physical challenges were many. Throughout his recuperative time in the rehabilitation hospital and at home, David, with assistance from some professor friends, continued to guide the research of his students and post-doctoral scientists, so not a step was lost.

David worked in his profession for another seven years before he retired and we moved to the desert, a place we both love. Now, we are advocates for brain-injury survivors through my blog, "Surviving Traumatic Brain Injury," at survivingtraumaticbraininjury.com and through my radio show, "Another Fork in the Road," on the Brain Injury Radio Network at blogtalkradio.com.

One night after dinner, I laughed as I watched our friend and David try to put together three magnetic rods and balls to make a triangle using *only* his right hand. I laughed as his hand jiggled all over the place and the balls rolled away from him, and I laughed as our friend slapped my hands when I attempted to help David catch the balls. I laughed as I tried to do the task and found it to be nearly impossible, and David laughed with me. We all laughed and laughed. Laughter is how we get through this life in the Disability Lane. Without a sense of humor, the nightmare would be unbearable.

I think of our nightmare like a traffic jam. You wait patiently, or maybe not so patiently, but you wait nonetheless. In David's case, his "traffic jam" is his brain trauma, and it's going to take a *lot* of reconstruction of neurons and other brain cells before he maneuvers his way out of this jam. Patience is key.

And so, my nightmare goes on and on, but through it all, we will battle, and we will fight. And, we will WIN!

Donna O'Donnell Figurski, whose life revolves around traumatic brain injury (TBI), is a wife, mother, granny, teacher, playwright, actor, director, picture-book reviewer, radio host, speaker, photographer, and writer. As a brain injury advocate, Donna has published articles in many brain-injury-related magazines on the web; writes a blog called "Surviving Traumatic Brain Injury"; is host of her international radio show, "Another Fork in the Road," online on the Brain Injury Radio Network; is a speaker concerned with survivors of brain injury and their caregivers. She has written a completed memoir, Prisoners Without Bars: A Caregiver's Story, and is now searching for a publisher/agent. Donna resides in the desert with her husband and best friend, David, who had a traumatic brain injury in 2005.
donnaodonnellfigurski.wordpress.com
donnaodonnellfigurski.com
survivingtraumaticbraininjury.com

Chapter Thirty
My First TBI Lesson: When "Alone" Becomes "Lonely"

Elizabeth Keene Alton
Eugene, Oregon

I never experienced loneliness before my traumatic brain injury (TBI). Sure, I spent plenty of time being alone. My then-husband was a firefighter who worked at least 24 hour shifts that sometimes expanded into 48- or 72-hour stays away from home. At times I thought that was part of the glue that held our marriage together for 25 years; the notion that absence makes the heart grow fonder. Plus, the more nights he was gone made for fewer opportunities for a stupid fight to occur. However, that glue quickly melted away after my brain injury, and our 25-year life investment turned into a penny stock.

Many nights throughout my marriage, it was just my son and me at home, having Mommy-and-me time. I really appreciated the balance of my evenings with my son, and the time we had as a family. As my son grew older and became more independent, like when he could drive, I relished the evenings at home by myself. I was a busy executive, and evenings at home alone, in control of the TV remote, with a simple meal of a microwaved quesadilla and a glass of red wine, made my heart hum. Nobody was asking me for anything. Ahhhh.

In 2013, this all changed, and being alone would never be the same for me. While traveling with friends in India, I was ejected from a safari jeep while photographing a Bengal tiger. I toppled out, head first onto the road ten feet below. I didn't fully understand what happened until weeks later. I vaguely recall the jeep moving and thinking, "Oh crap." My girlfriend in the jeep ahead of me was alerted to my fall by the thud when the back of my head hit the road. I was immediately unconscious. I spent the next ten days in three different Indian hospitals, including five days in a crude ICU, and I did not understand the severity of my injury.

The fact that that my injury happened in India, lack of a full diagnosis and several snafus led to me traveling back to the U.S. alone a few weeks later. I was immediately seen by a neurosurgeon and scheduled for my first MRI. I was relieved to hear the doctor say I wouldn't need surgery, but was surprised when he said my brain still had active bleeding—and I should have never been allowed to fly home when I did. The moment that still echoes in my mind though, was when he told me my referring doctor said, "I was a bright lady and could afford to lose a few IQ points." I didn't understand the gravity of his comment right away, and brushed it off as a joke, but it started to hit home over the ensuing months.

He was a surgeon, but he didn't explain what my injury would mean for the long-term or what to expect short-term, only that I didn't require immediate surgery to relieve the swelling from my brain. The doctor said that I had suffered a subdural hematoma and a frontal lobe contusion, and I should feel lucky to be alive. That was all I knew. I was grateful to be alive. I stayed home the next couple of weeks and thought I had better get back to work before I ran out of sick leave. I felt tired, had horrible headaches and was terribly irritable. The superwoman in me thought I just needed to power through it.

I scooped myself out of bed and went back to work. I was trying to keep up on emails from bed, but had several departments and many employees I felt were depending on me to return. A few days into my return, after a terrible bout of confusion during a meeting, my boss sent me home. I tried to return to work two more times, but finally threw in the towel. My 20-year career as a non-profit executive came to an end, and within that same timeframe, so did my marriage.

These changes led to the sale of our family home, and a somewhat impulsive decision on my part to relocate to Eugene, Oregon where my son was starting college. I thought a fresh start as a single woman would do me good. I desired to be close to my son—not considering he would be fully invested in living life as a young adult, and probably would not be so interested in watching Lifetime TV with his rehabilitating mother.

More importantly, I didn't realize how my injury and the move would disrupt the human connections I was leaving behind in San Diego—those people who were such a key component of my former life. My workplace relationships, my friends, brother and mother were all hundreds of miles away now. This was my first foray into loneliness, and my first experience with depression.

During my marriage, I was frequently alone at night while my husband worked, yet never felt lonely. I trusted that my husband would reliably return after long shifts away with no substantial difference in him or our relationship, which he did, shift after shift, month after month, year after year. I felt a sense of security and connection: a bond that existed whether we were physically together or not. In this context, being alone allowed me to maintain the spirit of connection with someone I loved. We experience this same spirit of connection with other family members such as parents or children, or close friends, and some experience it with their relationship with God.

My connection to my husband was broken, and being "alone" now felt lonely to me for the first time.

For years, a close friend tried to explain this concept of loneliness to me, but I had failed to grasp it, but now I do. I regret not being more empathetic and understanding sooner. This friend had also spent many nights alone over the years. She had an enviable dating and social life and a solid management career, yet she dreaded her nights alone. Dating and keeping busy with work didn't equate to the type of connections I had experienced with my husband and son. Alcohol slowly took possession of her evenings, and she numbed her feelings to replace what she was missing. Although we each spent nights alone, I previously relished my time and considered it an opportunity to care for myself. At the time, I was secure with the notion that my time alone pre-TBI was temporary, while Tricia felt her alone time might be infinite.

The connection with my ex-husband was based on the experiences we shared, and the trust I had in our relationship. Our relationship broke up for a number of reasons, but one of the primary issues was an erosion of the trust that occurred after my TBI. I've come to realize trust is a major component of our close relationships, not just the things we immediately think of like fidelity, but the aspect of trust that sets the foundation to maintain the spirit of "infinite connection."

After our breakup, I was no longer able to trust that I wouldn't be lonely forever, and realized that I took some of my other well-established connections for granted: my mother, brother, friends. It was then that it dawned on me the distinction between alone and lonely. It wasn't as simple as the absence of another human's physical presence. It's the difference between the frightening prospect that alone might never end, versus trusting that it's a temporary state based on having the relationship currency to intuitively feel okay or even great when spending time apart or by one's self.

My move to Oregon after the loss of my job and marriage, took me over a thousand miles away from my best friend, my mother and many other close connections. The loss of my career and driving license made it logistically difficult to form new relationships in a new state and neighborhood. My battle with loneliness snuck up on me; then hit me like a ton of bricks that manifested into my first exposure to depression. I had extracted myself from the lives of most of the friends and family that cared about me, and by relocating, it wasn't easy for anyone to drop in on me. Thanks to the perseverance of those closest to me, and some of my own determination, I realized what was happening and began making a more conscious effort to go to them, to consciously start nurturing my connections.

My TBI journey has been filled with both painful lessons and silver linings. The lesson regarding the distinction between *alone versus lonely* has been the hardest. It's still hard, but in addition to helping me understand my own needs better, it has helped me gain greater empathy for experiences I think I understand, but don't (like my friend's situation). My infinite connection with her is one of the most important and supportive relationships I have. She's been sober for several years and in a happy relationship with a new infinite connection of her own. Yes, we can judge a situation through our own lens, but what really matters is the lens the other person is wearing.

Today, I try to pay greater attention to nurturing the connections I have, and am more grateful of how precious they are. I've become more appreciative of what's to be gained by investing even small efforts in developing new connections, not with the expectation of return, but for the simple reason that all connections have the potential to enrich each other's lives and limit the potential of alone feeling infinite for ourselves or anyone else.

If you are someone with a TBI, or know someone with a TBI, or someone you think might be alone or lonely, take a moment to nurture your connections. It will mean more than you realize.

Before a harrowing safari accident in India, Elizabeth enjoyed a long career as a non-profit executive in the bio-research sector and owned a management consulting practice for several years. Today, she's a TBI Survivor and learning to survive well. Her 25-year marriage and career both ended shortly after her injury, but a new life slowly revealed itself as she came to grips with her limitations, and is using the rewired circuitry of her brain as an ally, versus an adversary. Today, she resides in Oregon and devotes her time to healing, advocacy, working on a memoir, and abstract oil painting from the floor of her living room.

Chapter Thirty-One
I'm Fine

Ellen Shaughnessy
Lowell, Massachusettes

On October 27, 2015, my world as I knew it was thrown off its axis. An assault at work by a patient caused me to hit my head multiple times on the edge of a desk, and then the floor. In charge of a large medical center, I was a nursing supervisor who made numerous decisions every hour.

As a nurse, I had made all of the medical decisions in my family, but when this happened to me, who was left to make them?

My first four months of recovery were characterized by 24/7 headaches, word-finding issues, memory loss, both past and present, dizziness, and many other symptoms. The problem was I couldn't differentiate all my symptoms, and I told everyone "I was fine," except for a headache! Clearly my executive functioning skills were compromised. It was so hard for me to figure out how to find the help I needed because I couldn't think coherently, or remember if I had found answers.

The TBI tribe was a great resource for me. Also I realized that almost every state has a brain injury organization that is rich with resources. It was February 2016 before I started getting cognitive and vestibular therapy, and by then I was so dizzy I could barely go out as open spaces, and noise and patterns bothered me. I hardly ever went out alone, and I didn't drive for a long period of time, which for a fiercely independent woman was very difficult. It took even longer for me to accept that *I may never be who or how I was*. I now know that it is what it is, and it's okay.

Being a little mellower might not be a bad thing. I take time to experience moments, nature, and people more now. A year later, the headaches and dizziness are improved, I am learning planning techniques, respect for my body's needs, and how to combat the dizziness. I have good days and bad, but don't fight them as much, and just let it be most of the time.

I realize my journey is not as horrendous as others…but it is mine, and has been very difficult for me. I no longer say I am "fine" to those who know me well. Yoga, meditation, my loved ones' support, and my own determination are helping me to hope that someday, I will be "fine" with the new me.

I have been blessed with a wonderfully patient and loving husband who calls himself the driver of Miss Daisy. He does "one day at a time" better than I do. For those caregivers out there, I think the greatest gift you can give is be there when we need you, but have the courage to give us space to try and figure our new life for ourselves.

Until this happened to me, I knew so little about the aftereffects of a TBI. Education is key to achieving this. My greatest professional joy was when I felt I made an impact on someone's life. My goal is to continue that joy, and be able to help others to be "fine" in whatever that means for them.

What I wish more than anything else for other survivors is that someday soon it will be easier for them to find helpful resources, and that medical professionals will be more aware of resources for their patients.

Ellen is a wife, mother, grandmother and RN. Her interests are reading and traveling. Her "new" life, since an assault at work in October 2015 changed her world, centers around staying upright, making lists, and attempting to organize my days with humor, love, and being open to new possibilities.

Chapter Thirty-Two
Live Life Large

Emma Glover
Calgary, Alberta, Canada

Today, I'm going to introduce you to two people: Emma1 and Emma2, or pre-injury Emma and post-injury Emma. No, I'm not schizophrenic, nor do I have multiple personality disorder, but there is a medical reason for the two Emmas, and this is the story I would like to share.

The medical incident occurred in 2006 when I started having seizures, and after a long process, I was diagnosed with something called Arterial Veinous Malformation. A brain AVM is a birth defect where one's arteries and veins grow into a tangled mess, which is at huge risk of rupturing and causing death. My AVM was "weeping" or bleeding, causing seizures.

Because it was causing me grief so early in my life—I was just 33—I was advised to have it surgically removed. So, 2006 became the year of brain surgery, and I ended up having four brain surgery attempts. They finally removed the AVM on October 13, 2006, and yes, it was a Friday! But in order to remove the AVM without posing future risk, they had to cut back a branch on my Medial Cerebral Artery (MCA), which resulted in giving me a right hemispheric stroke. The stroke left me with left-sided weakness and a number of cognitive issues, such as short-term memory issues, massive fatigue, and slow cognitive processing speed. I spent a total of 19 months in three different hospitals; the last two were focused on rehabilitation rather than surgery.

In meeting with my psychologist in the third hospital, I learned of Emma1 and Emma2. He was trying to help me understand that I would never be exactly who I was pre-injury, but that certain traits and characteristics of pre-injury Emma would also be in post-injury

Emma. So pre-injury Emma became Emma1, and post-injury Emma became Emma2.

What good things did I carry from Emma1 to Emma2? I think there are three traits: Strength, Determination, and Perseverance.

I worked extremely hard to gain and succeed at the career I had in Human Resources. I graduated with a Bachelor of Commerce in International Business with Distinction from the University of Victoria. As part of my degree, I lived and studied in Japan, including surviving the 1995 earthquake in Kobe, Japan, which was not part of the curriculum. After graduating, I lived and worked in England for a year. Then I returned to school at BCIT in Vancouver to obtain a Human Resources Management Post Diploma, as by then I had figured out that I wanted a career in HR. After finishing at BCIT, I was the first grad of that class to land a job, which was at Union Carbide in Red Deer. In 2001, we were taken over by Dow Chemical. Then I was moved to Edmonton in the HR Site Service Leader role while still maintaining responsibility for Red Deer, and picking up responsibility for a Manitoba site as well as some global responsibilities. I loved my career and put a lot of hard work into it. I would say that my career was my work, my hobbies, and often my social scene. I am quite proud of the hard work that I put into getting and succeeding at this career.

I was progressing towards going on an international assignment, when I signed up for brain surgery instead. And that's when everything changed!

I have used that strength, determination, and perseverance to survive nineteen months in three different hospitals, where I learned to walk again and re-use my left arm and hand, which was and will likely continue to be the hardest achievement of my life. I received physical therapy, occupational therapy, recreational therapy, and cognitive therapy. I managed to be discharged from the third hospital on December 21, 2007, over a year after my stroke. And then after living with my parents for a year, as my husband bailed on me while I was in the hospital, I now live independently in my own condo, which I absolutely love.

Independence is the main area where Emma1 and Emma2 differ. I was a strong independent woman pre-injury, one who travelled to New Zealand and Australia solo upon graduating from university. Now, as Emma2, I receive all kinds of help. I belong to a support group at the Southern Alberta Brain Injury Society (SABIS). When I moved out on my own, I received assistance from a company called URSA, which helped me to live independently. An URSA worker met with me weekly to help me live my life as independently as possible. She would help me strategize, plan and enact daily living activities such as grocery shopping, getting around, and managing money. I have since graduated from this program, but still use the skills I learned from URSA.

Living independently is a huge success as a brain injury survivor. Many of my fellow survivors either live in group homes or long-term care facilities. I hope that someday I will be able to handle international travel independently, but so far Emma2 has travelled to Gabriola Island, just off Nanaimo in British Columbia for a week, but it did involve staying at a friend's house and was stressful to carry out. I often have to remind myself that I'm only nine years post injury. This October 13th I will celebrate my 10th brainiversary. I now celebrate two birthdays a year: my birth, and the date I survived my brain injury and started life over again.

The work involved in rehab was the hardest days' work I've ever done. I would have multiple therapy sessions throughout the day. Think of a university class schedule where every hour you go to a different class. It was grueling, but I was determined to recover as best I could.

Now, I no longer work for a paycheck, but I do volunteer at my local library as a career coach in their Career Coaching Program to try and maintain my HR skills because I'm worried about the ever-widening gap on my resume, and still hold out a glimmer of hope that one day I'll be able to return to paid employment. I also volunteer at my local senior's residence with their Adult Day Program, which I love. The clients make me smile, and I make them smile, so it is mutually beneficial. I love that they wear nametags so my short-term memory issues don't mess me up. They don't always remember my name, but they certainly do recognize me and greet me warmly. I enjoy contributing through volunteering, but volunteering doesn't fully replace the fulfillment I felt from my career.

Because of the stroke, nothing comes easily, so everything I do is a physical and/or mental workout. Some of the issues I continue to work on almost ten years later include:

Maintaining focus and not getting distracted. I can't handle multiple inputs of information at the same time, so I have to put in a lot of effort to focus on one thing at a time. My parents are great at this. My mum, especially, knows that we need to finish one topic, and she let's me catch up with my iPhone before we switch gears and discuss something else. Throwing several different topics at me quickly is a surefire recipe for disaster.

Short-term memory. Everything important gets logged in my iPhone. My memory is not reliable, so if it isn't in my phone, it isn't going to get done.

Time Management. I'm either very early or very late. I have a really hard time being on time. I can no longer drive, as I have "left visual neglect" from my brain surgeries. This means I don't see peripherally to the left from either eye. To get a driver's license you need 120 degrees of vision to pass. There is nothing I can do to make this vision return, and my annual vision tests confirm that the neglect is still there. I don't miss the act of driving, but I sure do miss the freedom to go where I want when I want without having to plan a trip. Using public transportation makes it difficult to be on time. I see many drivers on the road that I'm sure I could drive better than, even with my left visual neglect.

Social Sensitivity. I find it really difficult to be polite when I just want to scream at someone, and I just do not seem to have patience as Emma2. Honestly I'm not sure I had that effective of a filter as Emma1, but it is certainly worse as Emma2. If you ever want an honest answer to something, ask me!!!

Fatigue management. In the early months after my brain injury, I slept twelve hours a night and still woke up tired. Somewhere along the way, I started having major sleep issues, and after a period of only sleeping about four hours of restless sleep a night, I went to a sleep clinic, and continue to fight for a good night's sleep. Now I sleep between five and six hours a night so I still dream of having a good eight-hour sleep, but at least I can function.

They say it takes ten years for the brain to heal, and that it's a lifelong rehabilitation. I am happy to be alive and doing as well as I am, although I'd love to be even better. Other than these things, I'm still the girl I used to be with a new motto: LIVE LIFE LARGE!!!

Emma was born in Britain and her family moved to Canada when she was two. She completed her undergraduate degree in Commerce at University of Victoria and then followed up with a post diploma in Human Resources Management at BCIT in Vancouver. She worked for Union Carbide Canada Inc and Dow Chemical Canada Inc. She now lives in a condo in Calgary with her fat cat, Minou.

Chapter Thirty-Three
Struck Down, But Not Destroyed

Erynn Adle
Traverse City, Michigan

People like to tell us how our brain injuries affect us. They inform us of the things they think they understand: how difficult it must be, how sorry they are, and how they are sure it will work out for a "greater good." They downplay our injuries because they don't understand them. They do try, shaking their heads, nodding along, adding in a somewhat stupid comment that makes them sound like they comprehend all the complexities of the human brain. But despite everyone's attempt to get inside our heads, *we're the only people who know what life is truly like with a traumatic brain injury.*

There was no blood, no horrific car accident, and I didn't even lose conciseness. I was doing what I love the most, correction: loved the most. It was May 30, 2015. My high school softball team was in Marquette, Michigan for our end-of-the-season district championship. We were getting smoked seven to zero, and the weather was ridiculously cold. The ball field was set up in the middle of a neighborhood, so in order to keep foul balls from flying into the street, a stretchy netting was suspended over the batter's box.

You may be wondering how this relates to a head injury. Little did I know that I would be asking myself that question for the next fifteen months of my life. I was up to bat, and trying my hardest to just get a base hit. I remember it all so clearly, which is probably the most terrifying part. I watched the pitch from the moment it left the pitcher's hip: a perfect strike. My bat came around through the zone *and I made contact,* just not soon enough. The next split second makes my heart drop every time I think about that foul ball flying up into the netting, which sent the ball straight back down and into the back of my head. My neck snapped down and my mind went blank. I can still hear the whole crowd gasp the moment after impact. I took the hit on the lower, right part of my head. I finished out the game and rode the most torturous five-hour bus ride back home.

Because I was wearing a helmet, didn't fall down, or lose conciseness, I was diagnosed with a mild concussion, and told that I should be back on my feet in a day, maybe two at the most. Nobody ever mentioned the eight weeks of cognitive speech therapy, or the twelve of physical therapy, or the fifteen months of headaches and dizziness. And, especially those forgetful moments I casually laughed off as being no big deal. I knew what was causing me to forget, but nobody else did. Nobody else knew why I wasn't the same energetic, 17-year-old girl I used to be, and no amount of explanation could ever take away the confusion in their faces.

My thoughts about what has happened to my life over the past year seem to change constantly. One week, I like to pretend it never happened. The next, I'm telling myself some big motivational speech about how all of it formed who I truly am. But the truth is, I am different now. I see things differently, I feel things differently, and I live my life differently than I did before.

Not being able to "showcase" my injury drove me crazy. The feeling that I needed to prove to people just how severe my concussion was, made my life miserable. I found myself jealous of people who had big casts or had had surgery. People believe stitches, surgeries, car crashes, and amputations. Apparently our "headaches, like all the time" don't show.

Life doesn't hit us the same way, and sometimes that seems unfair. But the truth is, we all get hit. After taking many Excedrin Migraines pills, and a few spoonfuls of reality, I realized that maybe it's okay that people can't see my injury. Even though they will never understand what it's like to live after a brain injury, I *will never know how not to.*

I learned to adapt to a new way of living, one where I can't watch television for more than an hour, or that I need at least ten hours of sleep to successfully get through the next day without a terrible headache. This is a life where my head comes first, and everything else comes second. I learned how to take care of myself, and inadvertently learned how to care for others.

I look back at the time I spent sitting in the smallest room of the hospital with my speech language pathologist who was asking me to start at one hundred and subtract in increments of seven while playing what should have been a mindless card game. I think about every physical therapist, chiropractor, craniosacral therapist, and doctor that has asked me the same questions. I've ranked my pain— on a scale from one to ten, ten being the worst pain you could imagine— probably 1,000 times.

All the hard stuff, like throwing up from being dizzy, wearing funny goggles to measure my heads rotation, it all gets forgotten, because I'm not the only one. I'm not alone. Everyone gets hit, sometimes we see it, and sometimes we don't. Getting hit with that ball took my life from its peak to the darkest times I had ever faced.

I will not preach about how getting hit was a gift, and if I had to do it over, I would because of the fantastic lessons I learned. That's not real. If I knew what was going to happen that day, there's no doubt in my mind that I would not walk out onto that field. But the reality is that it did happen, my world was turned upside down, and everything I once was sure of was gone.

I can't say I have it all figured out, because I'm far from that. However, I do know that whether we get hit and the whole world can see, or we get hit alone, we all suffer. As long as we all fall down, we might as well find a way to get back up again.

Now my senior year is under way, and I will be training for the best softball season yet. Missing my junior year lead to a lot of tears, but those tears have turned into motivation, and I am more than ready to step back in the batter's box.

Living and enjoying Northern Michigan's endless beauty, Erynn Adle is a Traverse City native. She enjoys most of her time outdoors, running, going to the beach, and playing softball. Graduating from high school in the spring of 2017,

Erynn plans to go on to further her education by studying Speech Language Pathology, specializing in brain injuries. Most importantly, she loves her family more than anything, and is incredibly thankful she has been blessed with them.

Chapter Thirty-Four
Almost Dying Saved My Life

James Manning
Huntsville, Alabama

Do you remember when you learned the date of your birth? Probably not. Similarly, I do not remember when I learned the date of my injury that had erased my memory. It was April 26, 2015, when I was 23 years old.

My earliest memories are not of being young at home with my family, but of being confined to a wheelchair in a hospital in Atlanta, wearing glassless frames with the left eye taped over. When I removed my "glasses," I had a most disorienting double vision. I was literally restrained in the wheelchair with a locking seatbelt. If I needed to use the bathroom, I had to call a nurse to unlock my seatbelt, and she would help me to the bathroom. Also, I had to call a nurse at night to unlock my seatbelt, help me into bed, and lock me into the seatbelt attached to my bed. Of course, I also had to call a nurse in the morning when I woke up. It sounds embarrassing, but it's just how I came up. I didn't know any better.

Eventually, I figured out—after being asked numerous times every day—what it meant when I looked for the nearest calendar to recite, "It is May 22, 2015. Today is Friday. I'm in Atlanta in the Shepherd Center." I had been moved there after already spending two weeks I do not remember at Huntsville Hospital. I had crashed while downhill skateboarding just outside of Scottsboro, Alabama, where I hit a boulder at high speed. My friends who called 911 say I was very drunk, but still sensible enough to wear a helmet. I was taken by helicopter to Huntsville because the crash collapsed my lung, and induced a coma caused by the same kind of head trauma that killed NASCAR's Dale Earnhardt, Sr. Once, while my mother was in the room, someone at Shepherd asked me where I live. I responded saying I lived in Auburn, Alabama, the town I had left when I graduated Auburn University two years prior. My mom was visibly upset at my answer so I knew it must be wrong. Now this prompted some heavy thought. Where the hell did I live? All I could really remember was the hospital. Whoever asked the question had insinuated I didn't live in the hospital, so I said the first thing that came to mind.

I stayed busy, sleeping a lot, but also with therapy. My parents or some friends came to visit every day. I healed quickly. I was only in the wheelchair for a week, and I left the Shepherd Center one week after they freed me from the chair. I was happy to leave. My therapy was getting less challenging, and sometimes I got weird looks from other patients when I strolled into the therapy room.

Upon leaving, I was able to remember that I had been a successful chemist in Huntsville, Alabama. The weird thing about my pre-injury memories, though, is that they did not feel like mine. I knew they must be mine, though, so I figured after leaving the hospital, I'd go about everything almost exactly how I used to, except now doing it with double vision. My doctors even said that it was possible that the double vision would go away, and that my mental fatigue would be less and less over the next year. No big deal...I used to frequently drink myself into a similar state.

After leaving Shepherd, I continued outpatient therapy in Dothan, Alabama, while living with my parents. It's a good thing that I stayed there for two months because it was apparent to me that I was not ready for the real world. I was very confused at living in an environment that was not designed for brain injury patients. I was still spending most of my time napping. Navigating my busy sleep schedule made it difficult to do anything, and, if I wanted to leave the house, I had to have a bailout plan in case the need for rest struck suddenly. In fact, I still find myself with a constant worry that I'll fall asleep at an inappropriate time.

After I finished my outpatient therapy, I moved out and quickly returned to work in Huntsville. My desire for independence was too great. I've determined from talking to my colleagues that I might have been reckless in coming back so soon. According to them, everyone was really worried about me when I came back because I seemed so out of it. However, I think returning to work was the natural course of my therapy. It was difficult returning to work and returning to living alone, but that's what makes good therapy. Good therapy is difficult.

So now I'm over a year out from my injury, and I think my injury can very easily be spun as a positive effect on my life. The frequent napping has stopped, but it has been replaced with insomnia. The double vision remains. The confusion has subsided a little, but still remains. My pre-injury memories have kind of returned, albeit in much less detail and with no real structure or order. They still don't feel like my memories, but they're *how I know my life has improved*. Before I got hurt, I was an alcoholic and drug user. In the months before I got hurt, driven by a good friend's fatal overdose, I pushed my consumption to extremes. I reasoned, "We're all going to die one day. Why not enjoy our time here?" However, I was not enjoying myself. My friends noticed, and one even told me he was happy that I got hurt while drunkenly skateboarding, as opposed to crashing a car or something else awful as he feared might happen.

The brain trauma gave me the perfect reason to turn my life around—*almost dying* saved my life.

When I was locked in a wheelchair in Atlanta, I started to come to terms with being locked up forever. Even though it was for just a week, it was all I knew. When they let me out of the chair, I could start to see my horizons expand. When they released me from the TBI ward, and again when I moved out of my parents' house, I was elated. This was much more freedom than I had imagined. My parents were told I might not survive through the night when I was first injured. Then they were told I might be a confined to a hospital bed forever. When I woke up, they were told I might not walk.

Living on my own was much more than anyone had imagined. I figure I should keep this trend going, of doing way more than was ever imagined possible, so now I've planned a month-long trip to Australia in October, and I am going to hike the entire Appalachian Trail next year. I also decided it's time to realize my dream of being a Ph.D. chemist, so I'm also applying to graduate school.

If there's one thing that I want people to take away from my story, it's that we're all capable human beings who can do anything we want. A colleague told me once that everyone in our lab is really inspired by my rebounding from this injury, setting my goals among the stars, and executing a plan to achieve them. I'm happy to be living, walking, proof that it is worth it to power through hardship. Don't feel trapped in any situation. Opportunities come from nowhere, and they're always disguised as hard work. Sometimes they're even disguised as traumatic brain injuries.

James Manning is a chemist in Huntsville, Alabama who was participating in one of his favorite activities at the time of his injury. As a result of his injury, he has decided to follow his dreams and travel the world. James is preparing to hike the Appalachian Trail and attend chemistry graduate school.

Chapter Thirty-Five
I Hate What Happened to You — But it was Bound to Happen

Jane M.
Richmond, Indiana

How many times have I thought, "It was bound to happen," since our son's accident? We despaired over our son's bad life choices and risky behavior for more than a decade, agonized over his latest relapse and blamed ourselves, begged him to get help for his escalating drug problem. Finally after the angry outbursts, physical violence, and theft of money, jewelry and expensive tools became more than we could take, we gave him the ultimatum—go to rehab or go someplace else, you can't stay here anymore.

So after a couple of weeks of couch surfing, he ended up at a friend's where the unthinkable happened. Somehow he fell down their basement stairs, landing face down on the concrete floor. Thankfully they called 911 immediately, and he was first transported to the local hospital, then taken to the trauma center in the city.

We had hardly slept since he had left, wondering if he was okay, was he hungry, did he call the resources I had given him to get help. But this was nothing new, and is the reality of having a drug-addicted son. When we got up on a Wednesday morning, my husband saw a missed call on his phone at around 1 a.m., "unknown caller." We looked at each other and didn't say anything, but saw in each other's eyes the bad feeling we both had. I got ready and left for work, and my husband left shortly after. Around noon he called my cellphone with the terrible news. I pretty much went into shock, but managed to drive home. We then drove the 100 miles to the trauma hospital.

Seeing him in the Neuro ICU comatose, all the tubes and ventilator, bruised, bloody and broken, was the most heartbreaking thing a mother should ever have to see—except him in a morgue. I kept telling myself that he's not dead…he's not dead. After we met with the doctors, nurses, and the social worker, we began to understand how grave his injuries were. Multiple skull fractures, orbital blowout fracture, and shear injuries intracranially. Ironically, the toxicology screen was clean except for a high blood-alcohol level. He was either too broke to buy drugs, or was trying to clean up on his own.

The neurosurgeon placed a monitor that was screwed into his head to make sure the pressure didn't become too great, or else they would have to cut a hole into his skull to relieve the pressure. He was on a 24-hour video EEG to see if he was having seizures. Then he developed pneumonia and had a bronchoscopy to clean out the lungs. His fever at one point was 106 degrees so they packed him in ice. He had neuro checks every 15 minutes, but remained completely unresponsive. I stood at his bedside and held his hand for hours at a time, talking to him, praying, pouring rivers of tears on him, until the EEG tech appeared at the doorway one night and very nicely asked me to move because I was blocking the telemetry.

My husband and I decided we would tag team at the hospital because there were no accommodations other than recliners in the waiting room, which was so crowded with people basically camped out for the duration of their loved one's stay. I saw pizza delivered there on more than one occasion. I did not want to leave his side even for a moment, but it soon became evident that was not realistic. So my husband took a leave of absence from work, and I filed for intermittent Family and Medical Leave (FMLA), not knowing how long our son would be hospitalized, or even a firm prognosis for his recovery. "Wait and see" is all we got from the neurosurgeon. We saw many come and go in that ICU, like the man in the next room just a little younger than our son, paralyzed from the neck down from a car accident; the girl who dove head-first into a pond and broke her neck; the beautiful Japanese lady whose mother had a stroke; stricken-looking parents and spouses; entire families filling the tiny rooms to say their goodbyes.

We drank coffee from the vending machine and brushed our teeth in the bathroom down the hall. Thus began our daily grind which lasted more than a month, driving the hundred miles to the hospital, spending a little while together, then relieving the other to go home for a shower, rest, and a hot meal. After about a week, I was at home doing laundry and got the call that he finally opened his eyes and gave the nurse the peace sign. Finally a glimmer of hope in what had been the longest and most painful week of my life. I fell to my knees and cried out to God, thanking Him for His grace and mercy and forgiveness. That's when I knew what I had to do—the very same thing—show grace and mercy and forgiveness. God is showing me what I need to do, and I have no choice. At that moment, I was so filled with such gratitude that my son's life was spared that all the anger and disappointment I felt towards him was gone. Instead I was filled with hope for a new beginning for him.

He was out of the acute phase so was moved to another floor for a week, then to an acute rehab hospital. He was very confused and cried a lot, was incontinent, and he had no short-term memory and iffy long-term memory. How much of that was from years of drug abuse, I don't know. Once he began to get his wits about him, it was clear this was going to be a rocky road. He became depressed and withdrawn, refused to participate in therapy, demanding to go home. I met with the social worker for discharge planning, and tried to find out what resources we might have to help him. Since he was still incontinent, and he wasn't safely walking on his own, I didn't feel our home was going to work.

That whole process was extremely frustrating. Handing me a bunch of pamphlets on TBI *is not* what I would call help! Finally, in frustration I asked her if he didn't have wonderful parents who loved him very much, what would happen to him? Her reply was that she would contact a homeless shelter and attempt to get him placed there. I was stunned. So of course we brought him home. His only real physical deficient was facial paralysis due to the facial nerve being severed from one of the skull fractures, and deafness in that ear.

Our life since he came home from the hospital has been a whirlwind of therapy, appointments with specialists, and surgery on the eye that wouldn't close. He is also on probation for a drug arrest prior to his accident, so we are having to deal with that. He can't drive, and finds no pleasure in anything. I remain hopeful that he will improve. His depression is long-standing, and is probably why he used to drugs as a way to self-medicate. The psychiatrist has made some changes in his meds so we will see. He remains drug free, and says he never wants to go back to living that life.

I want him to learn a new way to live, which may be the hardest thing he has ever done. He has a four-year-old son who lives in another state, and I hope that will be his motivation to get better and be a part of his son's life. He certainly wasn't able to before, messed up on drugs like he was.

I always pray on my way to work in the morning, and my prayer always begins with thanksgiving that my son is alive and mostly whole. I will never give up trying to help him get better, to learn to live a new way that's not centered around getting the next high. I want him to be glad to be alive, to be a good father to his precious little boy, to realize how lucky he is to have another chance.

In the meantime, my husband and I are finally going away for the weekend, the first time in eight months, to get away and breathe, and just be together as a couple—something we need to do for ourselves and our marriage. We can't take care of him if we aren't taking care of ourselves. I can't predict the future for our son, but stubbornly refuse to accept that the way he is now is the best he is going to get.

I myself am a work in progress, I believe all of us are, TBI or not.

No bio provided.

Chapter Thirty-Six
Road Bicyclist — Wear a Helmet

Jeff Squires
Mesa, Arizona

I have zero memory of what happened because I do not remember the weekend. The following is based on eyewitness accounts, facts from Mesa Police Department's Incident/Investigation Report, and family accounts.

I was riding my Marin Road T3 Pro Bicycle solo down Eagle Crest Drive in Las Sendas Mesa, Arizona on September 30, 2012. I was riding properly in the bicycle lane. A Camry-type vehicle went by me fast and close, and I flipped over the handlebars and landed on my head on the concrete at about 30 mph. The car did not stop, and the eyewitness could not swear in a court of law if the car had hit me.

I was lying on my side, blood shooting out of my nose, unresponsive, breathing very heavy and raspy. The eyewitness placed a blanket over me and called 911. The eyewitnesses were a mother and daughter on their way to church. A year and a half later I met a guy at the gym who had ridden by the accident scene and remembered seeing me, and he didn't think I would make it.

I was transported to Scottsdale Osborn in extreme critical condition with a skull fracture, sinus and mandible fractures, and L-1 spinal fracture, and brain bleeding. I was unconscious for five weeks, but not in a coma or induced coma. My kidneys shut down, and I had severe blood clotting. I had a feeding tube, tracheotomy, and my teeth were hardwired together to prevent losing them. I will never know what all I went through, but it was recorded on twelve CDs of medical records. I think I woke up a few times and pulled the tubes out of my body. I had a body brace on 24/7 for 15 weeks.

I do not remember waking up. Again, these are family accounts. I did not know what year it was. They gave me a walker, and I said, "Get it out of my way before I trip over it." I told the doctors, "I will not be here for Thanksgiving." They said our statistics indicate you will. When I said I am not your average over-eating soda-guzzling patient, the doctors said, "We can't argue with that."

I was released November 14, 2012. I went through physical, occupational, and speech therapy at Osborn and Health South when released. I had to take a neuro-psych test and a special driving test. I have PTSD now.

I contacted the eyewitness, and we had coffee and keep in touch. I went back to Scottsdale Osborn a few times to thank the staff. On my last visit, I told them they did okay, but what happened because I used to look like George Clooney. I took 364 days off from bike riding. I eased back into it by riding around the neighborhood. I had no fear because I had no memory of the accident, but I was safer than all other riders. I again became an A-group rider going on 70-mile rides averaging over 20 mph.

Going to work one day I saw a woman bicyclist by the roadside being worked on by paramedics. I stopped, stared, and as my eyes flashed, for less than a second, I saw me lying there. I cried and almost fell over. At a Starbucks recently, I saw some Mesa Police officers. I stopped and told them about the accident and their department's help in saving my life. One of the officers said, "I was the officer on your scene," and we both smiled.

Last December a friend went down on his bicycle, with no car involved. He was wearing a helmet, but he hit his head and died. I have not been road bicycling since.

Now I'm involved with the Brain Injury Alliance of Arizona. Through them I have started a bicycle helmet donation program, and received an award from the Mayor of Phoenix Greg Stanton.

As a TBI survivor, it happened and I cannot change that. I turn the negatives into positives and became a better person.

Jeff Squires is a TBI survivor from a near-fatal car/bicycle accident September 2012. Jeff sees himself as a better person since the accident. Jeff volunteers at Southwest Wildlife Conservation Center in Scottsdale, Arizona, preserving native mammals. Jeff is a University of Southern California Trojan fan. Fight on!

Chapter Thirty-Seven
Take a Walk in My Shoes

Jennifer Reaid Goodman
Cullman, Alabama

I am *a twenty-one year survivor*. My TBI occurred in a car wreck January 5, 1995. I was a fun-filled nineteen-year-old with lots of energy. I weighed about 116 pounds, and I was always complimented on my smile, long hair, and beautiful blue eyes.

This horrid night took it all away in a flash. I got in a 1993 Corvette with a friend. She was drunk, but what could happen to me? I was the passenger who didn't wear a seatbelt. We were recorded going 130 mph. They figured that speed from the skid marks and the multiple times the car was flipped, not to mention that I was thrown out onto the side of the interstate. A police officer was at my side in minutes. I had blood coming from my mouth. The officer had taken a class on emergency accidents, so he pulled out his Bic pen and punctured my trachea. He began breathing for me. I was airlifted to Carraway here in Alabama.

I suffered a punctured lung, broken collarbone, broken ribs, tracheotomy, broken jaws, broken pelvis, my right arm was only half way attached, and TBI. I stayed in a coma thirty-one days, with my momma by my side every day. When I did wake, I felt I knew what had happened. I couldn't talk because of the trach in my throat, and was really incoherent due to all the meds in my veins.

They transported me to a rehabilitation hospital. I was scared, and begged and cried for my mom not to leave, but she had to go. Every day I had different therapies to attend: Occupational therapy, physical therapy, speech therapy, and regaining strength. I couldn't walk, or talk, I could only whisper.

I was so tired after a few classes, I would sleep through the whole lunch hour, instead of eat. I stayed about a month, and upon leaving, I could walk again, but not real well.

Once home, my mother had to feed me, and hold onto me wherever I tried to use the bathroom. I mostly remember this neighbor mowing his lawn. The sound would hurt my ears so bad, and then the anger came—unremarkable, evil, mean anger, and over a lawnmower at that. So my mother thought a pet may help me soften up. I got the cutest little kitten, but I hit it and threw it down, so needless to say, the kitten got a new home. Then four months after the accident, mom took me to the bathroom as usual. She pulled my pants down and blood was all over. Horrified, I start crying. I had not had a period since the wreck, and totally forgot about it. New for me was that traumatic events will mess up your period.

A woman from the TBI agency in Alabama come to our home. Such a lovely lady, she would take me to a local community college and work with me on the computers. Then therapy started, and every day I went for occupational and physical therapy, as well as pool aerobics. After three long years of this routine, I could walk, talk, and even straighten my arm that had been contracted as bent. I started getting things back together; at least I thought I was.

I did attend the community college for a few years, maintaining a B average. I also moved out into my own apartment, and bought a car. I was doing pretty well, as years went on I saw my faults and flaws, but just went on. I wanted a child so much, I thought my pelvis was healed enough to get pregnant. I was the happiest pregnant person alive. My water broke and here we go. I was in labor sixteen hours. After a C-section, I saw my baby just a second, and she was so very pale. They doped me up and took my baby to the nursery where they did CPR on my baby for six minutes. She had a seizure, and was sent forty miles away to University of Alabama (UAB).

Even after having a C-section, I drove the forty miles every day to hold her. They told me she had a Methicillin-resistant Staphylococcus Aureus (MRSA) infection that is caused by a type of staph bacteria that's become resistant to many of the antibiotics used to treat ordinary staph infections, like penicillin. I then learned that my local hospital had given me too many epidurals. After twenty-eight days, I could bring my healthy baby home.

I've had the most precious days of my life with that little angel. When she was five, she acted just like me. If I asked her something, and she didn't want to do it, she would change the subject, just like I do. As a little girl, she thought I acted right, so she did the same.

At forty-one, I still have a lot of trouble with mood swings, and terrible anger. My daughter has a hard time with my brutal honesty and my cussing over the littlest problem. I try new medicines a lot. As I have gotten older, things in life have become extremely hard, but I still try to cover it up with a smile.

My main point I want the reader to know about TBI survivors, is BE KIND, you have no idea *what its like to walk in my shoes.* You can't see a TBI—and very little is known about it.

Jennifer had a TBI twenty-one years ago when she was nineteen. She completed three years of college. She has a healthy, smart daughter, who is an empathetic and inspirational person. Presently Jennifer is writing a book.

Chapter Thirty-Eight
Helping Others Through Experience

Jeremy Schmoe, D.C.
Minneapolis, Minnesota

In the winter of 2009, I suffered a concussion downhill skiing with my friends. I was going off a jump that I had hit multiple times the week prior—the only difference was that the angle of the jump had been changed. This caused me to fly over the landing with my arms flailing backwards as I tried to bring myself back to neutral. Instead I landed on my back as my poles and skis flew into the air. I was lying there trying to catch my breath. The only thing I could think about was how badly did I injure my neck, and were my ribs broken?

I can't remember how much time had passed before I got up, but I ventured into the chalet and foolishly went back out and skied the rest of the day. I remember feeling a little off after the fall, and had neck pain for the next few weeks. I did not take time off from school, nor did I rest physically or cognitively—my body or my mind.

Irony is that I was attending Northwestern Health Sciences University, getting my Doctorate in Chiropractic, where in addition to studying chiropractic I had started researching clinical neuroscience and functional neurological applications for complex conditions.

From the beginning of chiropractic school, I was introduced to the teachings of Dr. Ted Carrick, who is the pioneer of functional neurological applications in chiropractic. Since 1979 the Carrick Institute has taught courses in 13 different countries and 36 cities across the world. The Carrick Institute offers an exciting program of study in Clinical Neurology. The curriculum is accredited by the American Chiropractic Neurology Board. The program qualifies learners to be eligible to sit for the Diplomate examination of the American Chiropractic Neurology Board. Eventually I would sit for and pass the exam, and start lecturing for the Carrick Institute after I graduated.

In 2011 I moved out to Portland, Oregon to learn from Dr. Glen Zielinski, a well-known chiropractic neurologist who has become known in the TBI community for his work with the severely injured professional snowboarder Kevin Pearce.

Things were exciting, I was about to graduate and start my own practice. When skiing at Mount Hood, I hit my head again and whiplashed my neck. I felt slightly dizzy after this hit to my head, and had some fatigue. This lasted for a few weeks, and then things went back to normal...or so I thought.

One day while at a seminar, I rode the elevator back up to my room, and as I got off the elevator, I felt like my body slammed back the opposite direction, and my legs went weak as I fell backwards, onto the floor.

I started feeling these same sensations after driving, riding on escalators, and elevators, and when I was lying in bed, I sometimes felt like I was floating. The symptoms would come and go, and eventually they stopped—and I was left with off-and-on neck pain.

When I graduated from school, I drove back across the country from Portland to Minnesota. When I got back, I felt like I was on a boat rocking and rolling around. I started to develop severe anxiety, a racing heart, headaches, neck pain, dizziness when driving, plus the same symptoms I had experienced prior to my drive. They would come and go, and some days I would have no symptoms at all, while other days I would lie in bed feeling like I was going to die.

Keeping the symptoms to myself, I continued getting manual therapy, and I started doing vestibular-based exercises and making changes to my diet, which included autoimmune paleo and gut repair protocols based on blood chemistry analysis. This information was learned from Dr. Datis Kharrazian and Dr. Brandon Brock.

I started my own practice in 2014, and pushed through these symptoms. I ended up losing 50 pounds from the dizziness and nausea I was experiencing. During this time I started a traumatic brain injury course through the Carrick Institute that addressed all aspects of brain function that can be affected with traumatic brain injury. Soon the word got around, and my practice turned into serving people from all over Minnesota who traveled to see me to get treated for their persistent post-concussive symptoms.

My symptoms were getting better, until the day after going to a friend's wedding with Erin, my new girlfriend and soon to be fiancé. While driving home, the road had started rolling left and right, and it almost felt like my vision went upside down. I pulled off the road and ended up not driving for a few weeks due to severe vertigo.

Erin finally told me that I was so bad off that I needed to get treated, so I made an appointment to be seen at the Carrick Brain Centers in Atlanta, where I was treated for nine days total over a few months. I started to get more stable, and I developed new innovative exercises for myself once I felt better. I gained weight again over about a year, and had off-and-on symptoms that I still experience.

Over the past two years my clinic, MFNC Brain Rehabilitation, has been offering care to patients with persistent post-concussive symptoms. We have implemented an intensive care model of seeing patients for up to two weeks at a time between two to three times per day using vestibular, visual, manual therapy, and non-invasive nerve stimulation to improve people's body awareness and balance post injury.

When I look back there is no way I would be able to help people the way that I do without experiencing the symptoms that my patients are going through everyday. Without the help of my fiancé, I would not be where I am at today. I am so thankful for having the first-hand experience of suffering a concussion and gaining the knowledge to be able to help people with these devastating symptoms that occur post injury.

Dr. Jeremy Schmoe is a chiropractic neurological rehab specialist, lecturer and owner of MFNC Brain Rehabilitation located in Minneapolis, Minnesota. He works with patients from all over the Midwest and the USA. He is an advocate for traumatic brain injury awareness and started MN Concussion/TBI support group for his patients. His website is www.MNFunctionalNeurology.com

Chapter Thirty-Nine
My Feisty Little Brain

Jessica McCarthy
South Africa

It was so warm and comfy. I had that delicious naughty feeling, like when you press "snooze" one more time on your alarm, and you *know* it's going to make you late for class. But the consequences don't feel real because you're half asleep and the bed is so soft and enticing. I mumbled to my mom, who inexplicably stood next to my bed, "I know I should be working on my thesis, Mom, but I just want to stay in bed a little longer...."

I had no idea, despite the nurses and my mom patiently telling me over and over, that I was in intensive care. I had dodged death so closely that the taste of it was still in my mouth. I had recently emerged slowly and painfully from a five-day induced coma, having spent five hours in the operating room while the brilliant plastic surgeon patiently pieced my face back together. I thought I was being lazy, still being in bed at this time of morning. I had no idea that I had been in that bed for days, with a dedicated nurse posted to watch over me 24 hours a day, and to correct my head position if it strayed even a degree from the angles the surgeon had carefully arranged me in. I had never even heard the words, "diffuse traumatic brain injury with severe axonal damage"—at least, not organised in a neat diagnostic string like that. Now those very words described what was happening inside my 23-year-old skull.

Years before, when I was 19 or 20, my car battery ran out because I had left the lights on. After trying multiple roll-starts, I finally got someone to jump-start me, and my car ground into life. When the middle-aged Dad-type who had helped me looked in my battery, he told me it was completely out of battery water. I didn't know what battery water was. I felt like such a stereotypical girl, not knowing how cars work. I'd never needed to know about battery water before, because my car had been working fine. Now I was suddenly faced with having to learn details about the workings of the engine. Imagine it had been more extreme. Say the whole car had broken down, and I was on a desert island with no mechanics around, with a bunch of tools I didn't know how to use. That's what it's like to wake up with a brain injury. You suddenly realise that you've been relying so heavily on an intricate and beautiful machine that you just took for granted would always work, so you didn't learn too much about where all the cogs and screws fitted.

You don't ever imagine someone could press *ctrl alt delete* on your brain. You don't expect to start again, at the age of 23, or any age.

The following months and years of rehabilitation were characterised largely by moments of, "Oh my gosh, I never even realised my brain was doing that!"

I had never thought before about my brain looking at words on a restaurant menu, translating them into imagined tastes and smells, communicating with my body to work out what it felt like eating, setting off a series of processes that resulted in a decision being made, and then ultimately telling my speech organs to order the meal for me, all the while filtering out the unnecessary stimuli of the piercing lights in the restaurant, the auditory peaks and valleys of conversations coming from the strangers at other tables, the rough texture of denim on my knees, and the whine of the background music.

If you had asked me what I was doing in that situation before my TBI, I would have just said "I'm having a meal in a restaurant."

But now, all of a sudden, the words on the menu didn't communicate with my body the way they used to. I looked at the letters, pieced them together. "Chicken." Okay, I knew what chicken was. I knew it was a white meat and I liked it, a long-term feature of my regular diet. But I couldn't connect with what chicken tasted like, what it would feel like in my mouth, whether my body wanted it. I couldn't even hear my thoughts on the matter that well, because the elderly lady with the green scarf three tables down was laughing, and the waiter was clinking glasses as he put them down at the bar, and the child sitting under the next door table had just sneezed, and Frank Sinatra was crooning, and the rain drummed on the windows, and my socks were suffocating my toes, and someone's phone was ringing and the words on the menu were pulsing in and out of focus and I could smell something spicy that I couldn't name and… and… AND… the word "chicken" didn't stand a chance. It meant nothing to me, in the frenetic world of that split second.

Now, four years later, some things are a lot better. When I was in hospital I couldn't read at all, because I was so dizzy that I couldn't focus on the words and so fatigued that I couldn't concentrate. But two years later, I went back to university and finished my degree. Six months after my car accident, I started driving again. Despite having to move back in with my parents for the initial months of rehabilitation, I now live completely independently, and the money paid out by the Road Accident Fund in compensation for my injuries has allowed me to purchase my first home. These improvements are wonderful. They help to keep my spirits up when the long-term difficulties rear their heads—because make no mistake, a "diffuse traumatic brain injury with severe axonal damage" doesn't just disappear.

Even now, four years on, I am surprised sometimes by discovering something new that my brain handles differently than it used to. I look pretty "normal" to people from the outside, but I still have a brain injury. Menus are easier than they used to be, but grocery stores are my Room 101 these days. I get totally lost and overwhelmed in their fluorescent lights, loud in-store announcements, and demandingly bright colours. There's also the brand names that are designed to jump out and seduce you, the mind-boggling choices, and the shopper behind you whose trolley keeps nipping at your heels.

Brain injury is an invisible disability that can even fool *me* into believing it's not there. Sometimes I buy into the illusion, and then I push myself too hard. I stay out too late, or cram too many appointments into a day, or forget that I need to schedule in a rest after a visit to the grocery store. When I forget, I pay the price. The cost is usually some combination of fatigue, irritability, and feeling overwhelmed, which, if I leave them unchecked, can quickly spiral into panic and despair, and a dangerous wormhole of an idea that my brain injury has left me "broken" forever. I'm still working out how to navigate the balance between accepting that I really do have a disability, one that will probably affect me to some degree for the rest of my life—and remaining hopeful that I will continue to heal.

So far, I've learned two major things about the human brain:
1. It is infinitely *more complex than I ever realised*, controlling things that are vital to my daily life even though I had never even noticed that they existed before.
2. It is a *miraculous self-healing machine*. One of the wisest of all the many doctors I have seen told me that no matter how much or how little rehabilitative therapy I did, my brain would heal at its own pace. I couldn't speed it up by working on it overtime, and I couldn't sabotage it by taking a break and letting it be. My truly brilliant neurologist explained to me that there are tiny proteins in the brain that walk up and down the dendrites at a rate of one millimetre per day, repairing any damage they come across.

So I walk a line. On one hand, I need to hold the diagnosis "brain injured" close to me, so that I remember to go a little easy on my expectations of my brave, feisty little brain. This paradoxical brain of mine, which causes doctors to do a double-take when they see my original brain scan and mutter about how miraculous my recovery has been, but which still battles to handle the demands of a shopping mall.

And on the other hand, I don't have to let it define every part of me. *I am not a brain injury. I have a brain injury*, and I'm learning to work with it, but it's not the whole of who I am.

Jessica McCarthy, age 28, is a South African actor, puppeteer, and voice artist. She sustained a severe traumatic brain injury in a car accident in 2012, just a few months before she was due to graduate from university. Although Jessica had always considered herself a writer before the accident, her confidence took a major knock when her TBI caused her to have language difficulties, and this is her first hopeful venture into writing again.

Chapter Forty
You Are Not Alone

Joanne Ritchey
Toronto, Ontario, Canada

In September of 2013, we went to mediation for my case regarding the accident. It was a very stressful experience. It amazed me how low they would go to blame the extent of my head injury—to they point that they brought up my marriage with my ex-husband. I have no clue how they found out that I was previously married, but they tried to insinuate that I was physically abused by him, and maybe he somehow hit me on the head at some point in our marriage.

Then, I was told that any social media that I had was going to be "frozen." I was not to delete anything I had posted up until that point, and that they were watching.

That infuriated me! I had nothing to hide because nothing I had done or had posted gave me any reason to be worried. This made me very angry. Thinking about it now, it almost felt like poison in my body. For months, on top of having TBI symptoms, I walked around anxious, angry, and sick.

Until one day, I decided that *this was it. I was not going to let them control me.*

On December 16, 2011, while shopping in a store, a sign fell on my head. Not my fault. I started to research head injuries online, and then on Facebook. After I read Amy Zellmer's *The Huffington Post* piece, I realized I am not alone.

I guess I should start from the beginning to tell you a little bit more about the accident. It was just before Christmas, and the day before my son's birthday. My husband, Lonnie, and I took the day off work to go to an appointment and to get some Christmas shopping done.

Of course the first store we went to was our favorite clothing store. I reached up to look at the size for a hoody, and the next thing I knew, everything went black. I was seeing stars, and everything sounded muffled, like I was underwater. Although I was blacking out, I remember covering my face and leaning forward, almost knowing that the pile of clothing in front of me would catch me if I fell.

Lonnie was to the left of me, so he didn't see the sign actually hit me on the right side of my head. He thought it might've hit my shoulder, and then fell to the ground. A man with his baby in a stroller was a few feet away, and saw that the sign hit my head. He asked if I was okay, picked up the sign, and said to my husband, "This thing just hit her on the head."

I was just coming to at that point, and felt instantly very confused, stunned and everything looked foggy. Lonnie asked if I was okay, and showed me the sign, saying that it had just fallen from the rack. I should also mention that the rack was hanging about 10 feet high on the wall, and the sign was about the size of my hand, but it was solid metal.

I continued to shop because all I could think of was Christmas is a week away, and my son's birthday is tomorrow, and I need to get stuff done. As I continued to shop in the store, as hazy as things seemed, the lights got brighter, the sounds although muffled, got louder. And even though I was on a shopping mission, I started feeling defeated. I couldn't continue…I just had to go.

When I found Lonnie, he was chatting with one of the sales people, telling him what had happened. He just kept apologizing to my husband and offered coupons, and as sweet as that was, it did not help the situation. I told Lonnie, "I can't do this anymore. Let's just pay for what we have and go." When we got to the checkout counter, I asked to speak to the manager who came over. I explained her the best I could what happened, and without getting into too much detail, she wasn't very helpful, so I told her I was going to contact the head office.

When we got home from shopping, I had to lie down and close my eyes, so I did. I woke up a couple hours later to try to make dinner, but still felt so heavy, and the room seemed hazy. Throughout the evening, Lonnie started to get quite concerned, and after the fact, he told me that he stayed up all night watching me just to make sure that I was okay. I decided to go to the hospital the next morning because I still did not feel right. When I got to see the ER doctor, he flashed lights in my eyes, had me walk a straight line, and then told me to take some Tylenol and rest because I had a mild concussion. I went home and rested. What does "rest" really mean to a mom? I wish he would have written down what he meant by rest. In this whole ordeal, I have learned the true meaning of rest. We had my son's birthday party planned for that day, but had to cancel it because I was just not in any state of mind to prepare and host a party.

For two months I was still recovering, basically leaving the house to go to doctors' appointments, and then coming home to rest. Six months later I started to feel well enough to start doing normal things, going out a little bit more, being social, and doing a little more around the house.

Ten months after the accident, I felt well enough to go back to work, but I did have to change careers. For many years prior to the accident, I was in early childhood educator, and because of the accident, due to balance issues and my (lack of) patience, it was not the same. I was not the same person, and I felt like I *could not* work with young children. So I found a job in retail warehouse, which I love.

After working about six months, my concussion symptoms started to come back. The doctor said it was normal because I wasn't resting like I was before when I was not working. I would go to work, and I would come home to rest. But that wasn't enough, so I had to take some time off at my new job. This has happened a few times since the accident, where I've had to take time off work.

Instead of my concussion symptoms getting better, I have seemed to develop different types of symptoms. My biggest struggle was not knowing what was happening, and thinking something was wrong with me—that I was going crazy. Finally, maybe the third year of my TBI, a new doctor addressed it as a TBI. They didn't know what was wrong with me, and figured I should be better by now. I kept going for test after test, being on medication after medication, nothing getting better and nobody knows why. Don't get me wrong I really appreciate all the doctors—but they really didn't know.

I am a true believer of things always happen for reason. I was asked to do a neurological assessment. The results showed issues with short-term memory, aphasia, severe anxiety issues, and possible PTSD. The doctor recommended I see a psychologist regarding anxiety and PTSD. It was very clear that this doctor had no knowledge about TBIs, and he could not relate whatsoever, but he was there to listen. And that was fine; I was just going to go through the motions. As I was talking to the psychologist at my first appointment, he had asked if I had ever done physiotherapy, and I said no, adding, "I don't really know what kind of physiotherapy would treat head injury."

He referred me to a physiotherapist who specialized in head injuries. In that one session with him, I was provided with more resources and hope about my TBI than I had received in the last four years. I took his assessment, and right away he said that he could help me. At that moment, *I felt hope*. In that assessment appointment he referred me to an optometrist who specialized in head injuries. In appointments with this optometrist, I went through two very long assessments. Then I was diagnosed with Visual Dysfunction syndrome; my depth perception is completely off, and my right eye does not work in sync with my left eye.

Normally when you receive a diagnosis that is not great news, you may feel down, disappointed or sad. Receiving my diagnosis from the optometrist and the physiotherapist *made me ecstatic*. I knew at that moment I was not going crazy—and that they were going to help me.

I continue to see my physiotherapist, and I'm waiting to get my prescription glasses and start my vision therapy. I couldn't be more excited. Even though right now I'm struggling each day, I know that there is a light at the end of the tunnel…I can actually see it. My doctors and specialists don't really seem too positive regarding these alternative therapies and treatments that I am pursuing—and actually still want me to go for tests and prescribe me more meds. I think I'm going to take a break from that for now; however, I don't recommend that for everybody.

For me, knowing what I've been through, and how I feel, and how my body has reacted, I need to take a break from the appointments, from the medications, and from the tests. I will continue my physiotherapy appointments because they make me feel good, and I will go to my vision therapy because I know it's going to help me, and I feel good about this decision.

I do have my family's support in my decision to pursue these treatments. Their support throughout this has been imperative. It hasn't been easy for them to understand. I have my little dog, my BFF Quiggley. He is not an official therapy dog, but he has been therapy for me. I have missed out on so many things, birthdays, school trips, and dancing with my husband, but my family has stuck with and supported me through it all. For that, I am so thankful.

This is where Amy Zellmer's story comes in because that day I was filled with so much anger. I was determined to fill my social media with as much information about TBI as I could. Maybe those lawyers could get an eyeful of TBI, and a glimpse of what I was really going through. I stumbled on her story in *The Huffington Post*. It inspired me to continue to research, and from there, I have come across many stories through social media. It has turned out to be therapeutic for me. Everything happens for a reason.

I have learned you may have moments of weakness, but don't give up. I've learned I have to listen to my body, and I have to listen to my head, and when I feel fatigue, I need to rest. I have also learned that I am not alone. Knowing that is half the battle. You are not alone, whatever your battle may be, you are not alone.

Joanne Ritchey is a wife and a mother to two boys, and on her good days, she enjoys baking and cake decorating. She is honored to be part of this book and has been inspired to write more of her story and experience in hopes of inspiring others.

Joanne would like to thank her family and friends for being supportive on her TBI journey.

Chapter Forty-One
I Had Always Hoped

Jocelyn Schwartz
St. Augusta, Minnesota

I was a happy-go-lucky girl with only a few months until college graduation, but then my world turned upside down. I was a nursing student about to graduate with my bachelor's of science in nursing. So being a patient in the hospital was very odd to me. I was used to being the health care professional, not the patient. A nurse named Julie called my mom, saying that I was in a bad car accident, and that they were going to stabilize me and get me to a bigger hospital. It was extremely bad weather that day.

Mom called my boyfriend of about four years to let him know. He said the scariest thing was seeing a priest right when he arrived. He was probably thinking, "Oh, this isn't good." I was unconscious for a few days, but then regained consciousness—and then the real world sank in.

I actually had a job interview in Hawaii set up at the time of my car accident, and obviously I would not make the interview. I had a severe traumatic brain injury along with a broken clavicle, likely from the seat belt, and also third-nerve palsy, resulting in my left eye being closed for about two months. I now wear glasses with prism lenses to avoid my double vision.

At first doctors didn't think I was going to survive, let alone go back to nursing school. After a year and a half, I was able to go back to nursing school and graduate with honors. I passed my nursing boards right after graduation. I couldn't imagine being anything but a nurse.

I honestly feel like the luckiest person ever. I do believe you get out of life what you put into it. I worked really hard during my twice-a-week occupational therapy and speech therapy sessions, but also did many exercises at home, which included wearing an eye patch. I learned not to take no for an answer, and to do my best each day. I try to view every day with gratitude.

I talked with my speech language pathologist the month I was going to graduate college. She asked me what I thought was going to happen? I said, "I had always hoped." She said I think that's why you are where you are.

Jocelyn Schwartz is a Registered Nurse from Elk River, Minnesota. She has learned hope is very important during TBI recovery.

Chapter Forty-Two
Injured Cop Survives Brain Injury

Jon Casey
Anoka, Minnesota

My traumatic brain injury occurred on a beautiful fall afternoon in 1996. I was not injured falling or being in a motor-vehicle crash. Nor was it from any sports-related collision. I was assaulted. A man attacked me with a large knife and a steel table leg. I was struck on the left side of my head with the table leg, fracturing my skull. The blow made a silver-dollar size hole, breaking off four pieces of my skull, one of which was driven into my brain. This assault was work-related—I was a police officer.

I've wanted to be a police officer since I was a boy. My parents told me that when asked what I wanted to be when I grow up, I said, "A cop." I imagine they assumed the next week I would say an astronaut and a week later a cowboy. But I never wavered, and proudly served my whole career of thirty years as a patrolman.

If you work that long in such a dangerous profession, injuries are expected. I had been injured several times, but not necessarily in ways people would think of. I received first aid for smoke inhalation after trying, unsuccessfully, to save a boy from a house fire. I was put on medication after fighting a guy who was positive for hepatitis C, and getting his blood on me. I also was on medication after dealing with a sixteen-year-old who had highly contagious viral meningitis, who died later that day. I even had urine thrown on me. Along the way, there were countless scratches, sprains, and bruises. Nobody likes to get arrested, and some fight back with all their might.

In those thirty years, I was never shot or stabbed, but on a beautiful Sunday afternoon I was almost killed.

On that September day, Labor Day weekend, I was dispatched to meet with a man about a domestic-related dispute involving a roommate who had moved out and "stolen" several items. Since the roommate was not there, I didn't request backup. Also, I knew the complainant, having arrested him before. Several times since that arrest we spoke and had developed a good relationship. When I arrived at his apartment, he showed me a list of the items, and demanded I get them back. I told him I doubted he would never again see the frozen meat and dishtowels that were taken. I tried to explain this was a civil, not criminal matter, and little could be done.

I left but did call the ex-roommate who told me what I expected. The items were hers, and he even owed her back rent. When I returned to tell him the news, I was somewhat relived to see him sitting outside, knowing I wouldn't have to meet him inside his apartment. When I told him he wasn't getting his things back, he suddenly got very angry and stormed inside saying, "I'll take care of her."

As I returned to my squad car, I looked over my shoulder, and will never forget seeing the apartment door flying open. He had a knife in one hand and the table leg in the other. I radioed for backup. He started to walk away from me, apparently to find and kill the ex-roommate. This was noon on a warm Sunday, about a half block from a park. A car was coming down the street behind him. Suddenly he rushed me, and I had a short moment to decide to shoot or not. I chose not to.

I was fearful of shooting, and even at close range, missing him or having the bullet pass through his body and hit an innocent person. This attack occurred before we had tasers, so I struck him with my baton, knocking the knife out of his hand. He swung the table leg like a baseball bat, striking me in the head. I know by the large bruise that developed days later that I brought my left arm up in an attempt to block the blow. Fortunately, I remained conscious and was able to fight back. We struggled in the middle of the street—me with my baton in my hand, and him still holding the table leg. I remember a lot of grunting as our faces were against each other. I was able to force him down onto the ground, eventually placing a handcuff on one of his wrists. Then the first of many cops arrived and finished taking him into custody. He was dragged away and placed in the back of a squad car where he eventually kicked out a window. Later, I was told he confessed that in his rage he had every intention of beating me to death.

I was kneeling, looking at the ever-increasing pool of blood, and instinctively placed my hand to my head. I was shocked to feel that the area had already swelled to the point that it felt like half of a grapefruit. There was a large gash that my finger fit into. As more and more cops rushed to the scene, I started to realize how seriously I was hurt. Being the senior officer, I felt the need to remain in control and give instructions. But when I spoke, the words didn't come out right. It was as if my voice was on a vinyl record…and it was skipping. As a child and young adult, I've experienced numerous concussions. After high school I became an amateur boxer and fought for many years. Getting my "bell rung" was nothing new, but at the same time, *I knew today was different.*

I was rushed to the hospital. My bloodied uniform was removed and my wife called. She was told I had been in a "tussle," and that I requested she should bring me a change of clothes. I recall stopping a nurse from cleaning off the blood from my face, telling her to wait until someone from the police department came and collects evidence. I wanted photographs taken because I was "evidence."

Only later did we learn how serious my injury was. The blow from the table leg blew a silver-dollar size hole in my head. Four pieces of my skull broke off; one was driven into my brain. During surgery, a small piece of my brain was removed, and my skull was put back together with twenty staples. As mentioned earlier, he and I had a pretty good relationship. He had been taken to the same hospital, and I was later told by one of the cops guarding him that he wanted to visit me and apologize. He explained I was the only cop he liked. Hearing this, I felt thankful he liked me. Who knows what would have happened *if he didn't like me.*

The ten days I spent at Mercy Hospital in Coon Rapids were life changing. I drifted in and out of consciousness and experienced many emotions—pain, confusion, humiliation, denial, pride, and more pain. My suffering pales to many who have been through so much worse, and I realize that ten days is nothing compared to the weeks, months or years some are confined to a hospital. During my week and a half I lost fifteen pounds. I had been training for the Twin Cities Marathon, and was in the best shape of my life. Already slim from all the running, this was weight I could not afford to lose. Soon after surgery, my family and I left my room to go for a short walk around the floor. I was connected to the morphine IV drip. I made it maybe twenty feet, but was so exhausted I had to stop and rest. I had been planning to run 26 miles in two weeks, but now couldn't find the strength to shuffle to the nurses' station.

Light, smells, noise…everything irritated me. I became very sensitive to things that had never bothered me before. When my parents would visit, I would dread the goodbye, knowing my mother would hug me. The smell of her perfume nauseated me. I made my wife promise to forgo any scents, even urged her to use non-fragrance shampoo. When the staff would enter my room to check my vital signs, which was often, I would try to breathe through my mouth. One of the male nurses must have bathed in the cheapest cologne he could buy. I was convinced he hated cops—probably because of a ticket he got, which of course he didn't deserve.

I was also very sensitive to light. Even with the blinds tightly closed, I had someone drape a sheet over the window. The worst pain occurred when my brain began to swell. The doctors even considered removing a piece of my skull to relive the pressure.

This one moment I consider the lowest point in both my hospital stay, as well as my life. I wasn't eating, but still needed to take several pills. With a nurse's urging, I swallowed a couple of green beans and then the pills. I barely made it into the bathroom to throw up. I'd vomit the little I had in my stomach and then scream out in pain. I'd heave again and scream. This cycle continued several more times. I was now completely exhausted, and collapsed on the floor. There I was in my hospital gown, still connected to an IV drip, laying on a bathroom floor with sweat running down my face. I remember placing my forehead against the side of the toilet. It was cool, and that felt good. A minute later I'd switch to the other side of the toilet bowl, soothing my aching head.

My relatively short stay in the hospital can't compare to what others have gone through, but still it was not easy. I dealt with a lot of pain, confusion, needles, waking up in cold sweats, and the nightmares. Luckily, I had a strong and loving family—and also, a desire to be a cop again.

Before being released from the hospital, I met with the surgeon who operated on me. He explained that no one could say how my recovery would be, or if I would even recover completely. He mentioned how much of the brain was not understood, and no matter how many CAT scans were in front of him, there was no way to predict my future. Unlike a broken bone, my broken brain would heal differently. Certain memories may have been lost, and my personality changed forever. It was hard for me to accept this concept. Was I now someone different? Sometimes it bothered me to think I might not ever be the same. Others times, it seemed like an incredible opportunity.

I was being given a challenge to become a different person, a better person.

Being home was incredible. I can't describe how it felt to finally be with my wife and teenage daughters, regaining my strength, and getting my appetite back. My wife had gone back to work, and my daughters went back to being high school kids, and I hoped they were not worrying about me. Everything was looking up, at least until the depression hit just a week after I was home. It came on fast and strong. Almost a physical pain, it was heavy, and it hurt. On days that I managed to force myself to leave the house, I'd drive to a mostly deserted, half-empty shopping mall. I would spend many beautiful fall afternoons walking around inside this dreary place trying to cope with all these new emotions. By this time, my hair had grown back so the scar was covered, and I was almost back to my normal weight. I looked fine. Everybody said so, but I wasn't fine, I was still injured. Often, as I walked through the empty mall, I wished I had a cane or crutches, maybe a visible scar—anything to signify I was still hurting. I remember limping once, for no other reason than to show I wasn't healed and was still very much hurting.

I kept the depression a secret. I knew I had people in my life who would have done anything for me. As a male and a cop, I guess I felt embarrassed to talk about it, that it was some kind of weakness. I certainly don't feel that way now. Fortunately, it didn't last long. But it was hard for me to understand what was happening. Another change…was the crying. In the months after my injury, I would cry. It felt good to have that release, at least when I was alone. Once, shortly before I was about to go back to work, I cried in front of the police chief. I was in his office and broke down. His response was, "Gee, I've never had one of my officers cry in front of me." I felt embarrassed and extremely humiliated.

That's when I started to realize how wide spread ignorance about brain injury is.

Three months after the assault, I returned to work, going right back to patrol. My uniform was still a little big, and I had some uneasiness about jumping back into the domestics and bar fights. But being a policeman again is what drove me to such a fast recovery. I desperately wanted to wear that uniform again. I couldn't stand the thought of not being a cop, and I did everything in my power to make it happen. However, I felt "uncomfortable" doing the job again that I'd done for so many years. I equated this uneasiness to having been gone for three months, but now understand it was because I was still healing—and that I went back to work *too soon*.

Only someone who has experienced a brain injury can relate to the feelings and emotions that I felt. As weeks went by, I could tell I was changing, improving. Occasionally, I would do a self-assessment. I'd ask myself if I was any different today than two weeks ago. I would feel different, and know I was still getting somehow better. Another two weeks would go by, and again I'd feel some change or improvement. It's hard to describe, but something just felt different from one week to the next. This happened for a full year during which I felt I was recovering, and in some ways I still am.

Finally, the day came that I felt the same and realized this was my "new normal." It happened about the same time as I was in the courtroom witnessing my attacker accepting responsibility, and being sentenced to eight years in prison. I met his mother, who also was suffering, and I realized how deeply affected others were besides my family and me. As he was being led away, I shook his hand and wished him good luck. He gave me an emotional and honest apology—and that was all I needed to go on with my life.

Since my injury, I've finished my college degree and also received a teaching license. I married off both daughters and now have four, soon-to-be five, grandchildren. I worked another dozen years as a patrolman and retired recently. I am so thankful to have survived that day. Unlike so many brain injury survivors, I got my life back. Sometimes I question whether I should have drawn my gun and shot him. Certainly, that would have saved me a lot pain and suffering. But I might have missed or the bullet could have gone through his body and hit a bystander. I don't think about it often. I am proud I held my ground that day and prevented anyone else from getting hurt. As a cop, my responsibility was to stop him, and that is what I did.

During those last years of my career, my perception of brain-injured people changed, certainly with those I dealt with on police calls. I learned that even though a person with a brain injury may look fine, he might not be. Sometimes I'm asked if I have any restrictions, or if there is anything I can't do now that I could before. My answer is that other than having to write things down, *I can't do any housecleaning.* I find it hard to vacuum or dust. Cleaning the bathroom is really difficult. I got away with this "limit" for a short time—and then my wife reminded me I never did those things before.

Jon spent thirty years as a police officer, all as a patrolman. He was brutally attacked and had his head fractured, receiving a traumatic brain injury. Within months he was back at work and continued working for another seventeen years.

Chapter Forty-Three
One Careless Driver Changed My Life's Trajectory

Julia Potocnjak-Overn
Tyler, Texas

My brain injury occurred in October 2013. I was stopped at a red light, and was hit from behind, causing me to hit the driver in front of me.

I was in my third semester of graduate school, and a teaching assistant at a charter school specializing in STEM concepts. After the accident, I was taking valium and driving to school in so much pain and mental fog—doing this so I would not fall behind. Two weeks later, I was having STAT MRIs and being referred to a neurologist. I went from being an athletic former personal trainer, to a person who could not get out of bed, feed or dress herself. I was traumatized by what had happened to my body and brain. I was angry at the driver, thinking: How dare this person hit the pause and reset button on my trajectory that I had worked so hard for!

Fast forward almost three years, and I have had every diagnosis from closed-head trauma to suspected aneurysm and pituitary cancer, dystonia and epilepsy, essential tremor and moderate cognitive impairments

I had to walk away from my studies and my job—I had to focus on getting better. I started doing less-is-more (LIM) yoga. I went to physical and occupational therapy for a month before I was told that in fact, therapy three days a week was making whatever I had worse. At that time, I was told most likely I had sustained damage to my frontal lobe in the accident. I tried to lift weights, even trying crossfit training for a time before it became too hot in the facility, and I would have seizures after the workouts. I started the keto low-carb diet to see if that would make a difference in seizure activity and energy levels. I was a very compliant patient and took all of the drugs I was prescribed. I got a cane to help with walking, and we moved from an upstairs unit to a downstairs one so I could finally take the dogs outside and gain back some independence.

I can't say how long my recovery will be because I am improving everyday, even if nobody can see it.

My biggest advantage has always been, and continues to be, advocating for myself. When I want additional testing or referrals, I communicate with my health care team until I get what I am seeking. I have asked for discount cards at the doctors' office to offset medication expenses. I asked for referrals to a top movement disorder specialist and neurologist over at University of Texas-Southwestern for additional diagnoses or changes in treatment plans. I advocated to see a therapist whom I meet with bi-weekly. I'm also thinking outside the box in terms of treatments. My mother purchased a bike trainer so I can work on balance and coordination. I do yoga both seated and standing several times a week, depending on how I feel that day. Brain fatigue and body weakness is another aspect I deal with, and nausea and migraines seem to like me a lot, too. In fact, nausea has become my worst best friend.

I would like to connect with brain injury survivors old and new by saying this: "Take every day as a new day to test yourself, to be good to your body and nurture your soul." I would like readers of my story to feel encouraged, inspired, and empowered. We are all resilient, strong animals. Being positive no matter what you are going through, helps the hard days seem a bit less difficult and the good days that much better! Think outside the box. Pick up an adult coloring book and get lost in it. Try a yoga class or take naps (you're allowed!). Volunteer for something you wouldn't normally. Survivors and caregivers need to reassure us that we are doing great! Life changes happen everyday, and we all have battles we are attacking from every side. Feeling alone? Connect with friends and loved ones, or call someone else who's close to you. Survivors who are dealing with depression and/or anxiety alongside their injury should not ignore these issues. There is still such a stigma regarding mental health, and I don't know why. I am taking anti-anxiety and depression medications, including Cannabidiol (CBD) oil. Make sure you are aware of and talk to your doctor about all of the treatment options available.

The world needs to understand this topic, and the invisibility aspect of these injuries. We are all still human beings, and shouldn't be discounted because of the handicaps or disabilities that are not visible. We are visual creatures that need to start paying attention to each other, communicating with each other and build up each other. Maybe your neighbor down the street has sustained several brain injuries over his lifetime, but is too proud to ask for help. Reach out to him. Maybe you know someone who has a child with a brain injury. Call and see how they are doing. *Caregivers of traumatic brain injury patients are also invisible, and they need to be taken care of as much if not more than we do.*

My hope for sharing my story is to inspire someone and get him talking—to his caregivers and to his health care team. My hope is that they demand more from their healthcare providers. Brain injuries are so complex, not clearly understood, and there is much more to learn yet. Demand more. We are the instruments that can steer our care and recovery in ways that can make positive outcomes so much more than we ever dreamed.

For caregivers, please be patient and understanding with us. So many things are going on with our emotions, thoughts, and our overall sense of wellness and being. We love you and appreciate you for everything you are to us. Please let us know when we are being pissy, taking advantage of you, or are being ungrateful for you. Caregivers, you make us accountable, make us recognize when we need help, and are our cheerleaders who call, text, visit or check-in with us because you care. And we love you for it. If our caregivers or loved ones are concerned about our medications or dosage, or suspect we may be abusing them, it's our job to hear them out. They are concerned about our recovery as much as we are. Will we both have bad days? Absolutely. Will we both have good days? YES. Finding humor in any situation is not a skill or talent, for me it's self-preservation. Making each other laugh while we celebrate another day is a gift we give each other.

Julia Potocnjak is a native of Canada and is also a mum to four fur kids, along with her chef husband Bryan. She holds a bachelors degree in Biology from The University of Texas Pan American, is a Mango Health ambassador and recently started working in an after-school program teaching STEM based activities to children grades 3-10.

Chapter Forty-Four
I'm a "Recovery In Progress"

Juliette Fiechtner
Fargo, North Dakota

My first head injury was in 2008. I was moving my 1-year-olds room around by myself when a suspended bookshelf fell on my head. It felt as though my skull had cracked. An emergency room visit, CT scan and message, "see your doctor if symptoms persist" were the outcome. I remember feeling ditzy and forgetful for about a month, and that was about it.

Fast forward to February 2016, I slip on some sandals to walk to the mailbox. I notice a patch of ice by the mailbox, and mentally tell myself to be careful. In a very Charlie Brown way, I slipped, and cracked the back of my head on the ice, and had it not hurt so much, I would've cracked up laughing. I went to my physician's office where one of the doctors said, "Yes, it's a concussion," gave me a pain shot in my tush and sent me on my way. I was going to school at the time, and found my philosophy class became very difficult. Open book tests, online at home, were a chore. Again, other than feeling slightly "off," I wasn't concerned.

May 20, 2016 I had stopped at a crosswalk when my car was rear-ended hard. Immediately I knew something was wrong. My hand went to the back of my head, and I sat in shock as my car came to a stop. When I exited the car, I found myself needing to sit down. This was my first car accident, so I didn't even realize my car should be towed. Finished with the police officers, I went to pick up my husband, because that's where I was going when collision occurred. I had him drive, and on our way home, suggested I should go to the emergency room, but he suggested urgent care, and by the time we got there, it was closed.

So, I went to urgent care the next morning, and the doctor there did a thorough exam, said it was a mild concussion, and I agreed. He told me to follow up with my primary doctor, and five days later, I did. Something was totally different about this concussion. It hurt more, I was foggy, couldn't find my words, and I could barely muster the energy to move. She sent me to physical therapy. I went, but a few weeks later I wasn't having improvement, so she sent me to a TBI specialist where my fate was handed to me: Post-concussion syndrome. That evening my husband and I had relations, and at the end, I knew it had re-shook my head. I woke up the next day in extreme pain and was very frightened. Thursday became Sunday, and I was supposed to be leaving for Hawaii on Wednesday. Monday I found myself wanting to go to the ER, which I did, and was told no flying, then, was given an IV of meds and fluids. *I wanted to scream.*

That was four months ago. I now have six different specialists, doctors, and therapists: 1) Physical therapist, 2) TBI specialist (speech pathologist), 3) Primary care physician, 4) neuropsychologist, 5) psychologist, and 6) neuro optimologist.

After 24 years as a stylist, I haven't worked since the accident, and don't see returning anytime soon. My career is essentially over. I have been told to put college on the back burner.

My symptoms include: word dismorphia, trouble accessing words, trouble sewing a straight line, head pressure, headaches, scalp tingles, sleep problems, reading problems (I used to read several books a week, now none), trouble concentrating, ear ringing, trusting my instincts, memory, concentrating, mild cognitive disorder, midline vision shift syndrome, light-and-sound sensitivity, and background noise challenges. These issues, to name a few, make it impossible to engage in a conversation, go to the store, be any place that is noisy or crowded or lit with florescent lights.

My goal is healing, so I have cancelled all work and two vacations. I also feel like my children have been robbed of their summer, my husband robbed of his wife, and me robbed of a normal life.

Most people don't "get it," and I've done my best to not make a big deal out of it. I rarely post on social media about my injury, because people don't understand. I did send my children to school this fall with letters explaining my condition. My husband has been amazing, helping around the house, taking the kids out. He admitted that he's had a few moments of irritation, but mostly he's been remarkable. Even my seven and nine-year olds have handled it well, because I have made each of them sit in when the TBI specialist talked to me.

Most recently my physical therapist has started using Keniseo Tape on my shoulder and neck, and I finally can feel somewhat normal. I am forever grateful that my physician sent me to the correct therapies for traumatic brain injury right away. I cannot imagine going through this without the right team to support me, educate me, teach me how to live my life in a totally different way. My speech pathologist (I call her the Brain Lady) has given me the tools to be able to cook and sew, and make it through the day without burning completely out, like, sew in stages, cook one thing at a time, use a timer, take naps, schedule everything.

It's a long journey ahead, but I can do this.

Juliette is married to her husband of 10 years, who is a pilot in the Air Force as well as flying commercial, and they have two boys (7 & 9) and live in North Dakota. She was a hairdresser for 24 years (20 years in Arizona), until a car accident in May 2016 robbed her of her career. She now spends her time sewing, painting, writing, educating herself on TBI's and going to therapy.

Chapter Forty-Five
My Son Ryan

Kathleen Whidden
St. Charles, Illinois

I'm a caregiver for my 28-year-old son. He acquired his brain injury eight years ago on September 21, 2008, when he was twenty and in college. I received a phone call at approximately 2:30 a.m. from Ryan's friend. I thought Ryan was in a car accident, but that wasn't the case. He was severely injured, and I needed to get to Edward's Hospital in Naperville, Illinois, as soon as possible.

The ride to the hospital felt like the longest ride of my life. Also it was very foggy, and I often couldn't see in front of me. I arrived at the hospital and went to the Emergency Room where I met with a chaplain. He tried to explain that this was very serious. I remember running past him to get to Ryan's room.

Ryan lay there unconscious, and not moving. Apparently, he went to a party that night and drank a lot of mixed drinks and beer. The police came and Ryan and his friends started to run. Ryan had already received an under-age drinking violation on campus. He decided to jump off a second-story balcony—and landed on cement.

Ryan's blood alcohol (BAC) level was so high the doctors didn't know at that point if it was alcohol poisoning or the fall that caused him to black out. After getting a CAT scan, the doctors discovered that Ryan had six bleeders to the brain and a fractured skull. A shunt was put in Ryan's brain to bring down the brain swelling.

My ex-husband and I agreed that I would stay overnight at the hospital. This was a critical time because if one of the bleeders bled, Ryan could die. I stayed next to him for several days until my parents came and I could go home for a bit. My friends had brought me socks and a toothbrush. I cannot tell you the agony I was experiencing. I couldn't even function.

Ryan woke up from a medically induced coma after three weeks. He had to learn how to talk, walk and do basic every-day functions. He went to Rehabilitation Institute of Chicago and stayed there for another two weeks. Ryan had to complete outpatient rehabilitation in Willowbrook, Illinois.

Ryan has been able to work part time. Several years ago, I hired an attorney so that he could collect social security disability, which he does. Not one of his doctors or social workers told me that I should do this.

It has been a long struggle for Ryan. He has problems with impulsivity, problem solving, and organizing. He's on three different meds: a mood stabilizer, an anti-seizure medication, and a stimulant. Ryan has also been diagnosed with bi-polar since his accident. If he doesn't take his meds, he will experience a mania that has landed Ryan in a mental hospital and a nursing home.

I pray every day that it's a quiet one. Ryan's personality has changed. He's quieter and not as affectionate as he used to be. It's been a rollercoaster ride for both of us. I know he gets frustrated when he can't remember something or loses his things.

Every day I mourn the old Ryan, but I have learned to accept the new Ryan. I love him no matter what, and try to tell him how good he's doing. It's a very difficult life for me since I'm a single mom, work fulltime and care for Ryan. I've lost boyfriends, friends, and have been warned at work about my absences. I feel for both the caregiver and patient.

No bio provided.

Chapter Forty-Six
The Lady "Bug" Begins to Fly

Kathryn Duffy
Clementon, New Jersey

My husband and I had been together five years, and married the summer of 2011. On a warm summer evening, August 18, 2012, my life changed forever. It was a beautiful Saturday, and we decided to take a ride to the farmer's market. We left our house around two, and ventured around the market. As we left the market, there is a famous chicken wing place not too far away so we decided to get some dinner. Before leaving I had to go to the bathroom. We always had an agreement that he drove to our destination, and I drove home. When I got to the car, he was behind the wheel, so I just accepted he wanted to drive because two weeks prior we bought a 2007 Cadillac CTS, which he had not driven much. I was getting used to the new car.

As we started our journey home, things were good. When we got to the road we live on, there is a curve and speed limit says 35 mph. But I was not paying much attention, and was singing a song (the title has never come back to me). As we took the turn, I suddenly realized he was speeding. He made the turn, but as he tried to straighten out the car, I felt it lift from the rear and head towards the trees on my side. I was buckled; he was not. It was like slow motion for me because I knew I was getting hurt.

The accident report said he was going 70 mph. I remember him pulling me from the car and sitting me down on a tree the car had knocked down. My husband was focused on me. As time went by, people started arriving. As I sat there waiting for medics to arrive, a woman sat down next to me. She put a rag on my head and said, "You're bleeding, please stay calm." When we got to the hospital, they did the MRI and discovered the bleeding on my brain. When I asked my husband who was the woman sitting next to me on the tree, he said, "What woman?" Through the traumatic event I forgot about the mysterious woman.

Immediately I was taken to Cooper Trauma Center—not knowing if I was going to live or die. I recall lots of people around me. Hooked up to every device, I was terrified. All I wanted was to speak to my son and my father. The care that I was given in the hospital was amazing. The doctor came in 24 hours later and said I was a miracle because my brain had stopped bleeding! He told me the recovery would be a long and frustrating one. I also recall him saying to me that *you will never be the same person*. I didn't pay him much mind because I was alive, and figured all this pain and suffering soon would pass, and my life would go on. I have been through a lot of health issues, and believed I was strong enough to get through this tragic event as well. They kept me 11 days, three in intensive care and the remaining days in a regular room with other patients. The symptoms had begun—the noise and the light and the spinning. As for the pain, it was horrible. My sternum hurt so much from the seatbelt, and my neck has many issues, too. My husband would work half a day, and then come spend second half with me. I really wanted to get out of the hospital and start the recovery process.

As I arrived home things began to settle in. This was my second husband. I have a wonderful son from the first who was seventeen then. I began living or existing in his room. My family stopped in, but truly did not know what to do for me. My husband went right back to work, and I was left to handle this alone. As the days went by, it got harder and harder. Weeks were full of depression, anger, light and noise issues, vertigo, and immense pain that I pretended didn't exist.

Then I realized...*the woman I knew all my life was not the same person. I needed care, and no one knew what to do.* My husband worked, came home and went to bed. I was screaming inside, not able to handle the fact that no one was getting how severe this TBI was. So although I was married, we apparently were not a team. I started figuring out how to get myself to the doctor appointments. My husband took me to one test and insisted I could make all my future doctor's appointments in the evening. What! My functions are the best in the morning. As the day goes on, I want to stay home and rest. I did my best to make him understand I was not the same person, and I needed help. All we did was argue, and at times it was physical, and his unkind words were unbearable. As we were driving one night, he said and I quote, "The next tree I hit, you will be dead." The strength in me was starting to build, and if I didn't do something soon, I wasn't going to survive.

On July 3, 2014 almost two years after the car accident, I quietly moved my things out my son's window and loaded my car. I told my son to meet me close by, and we headed for the woods, where we lived in a tent for six weeks. Even after finding out where I was in the woods, my ex never attempted to come help me. We finally found a house about forty-five minutes away, and I began to put my life back together again at age 47. A year later we divorced.

To this day he does not believe there is anything wrong with me. He didn't want to learn about the brain or even go to counseling. Everything happens for a reason. Hitting that tree and receiving this brain injury opened my eyes to his abuse and very selfish ways. I married him "in sickness and in health," and there was nothing I could do to prove to him I had a broken brain. Unseen injuries are the worst.

As my son and I began our new journey together, we both knew it would not be easy. A condo became available. He started working full time, and I stayed home alone…very alone. One day I was falling apart, thinking about horrible things like hurting myself. Never imagined this is where I would be. That was the day the light shined in my room. I decided to call a number the hospital gave me with one of three packets they sent home with us.

What needs to change is the part about caring for someone with a brain injury. People must have caregivers and people around them the moment they arrive home. These loved ones need to be educated and understand it doesn't just affect the injured; it affects the whole family. The number I found was Traumatic Brain Injury of New Jersey. Dialing that number saved my life! They found me caregivers, a new computer system, and support of people that know how debilitating a brain injury really can be. I started seeing therapists and having biofeedback every week. I could barely get there, but pushed myself through blurred vision and vertigo, and drove myself. I knew this is what I needed to make things better.

I had applied for disability benefits right after the car accident, and waiting for them to approve me was some of the worst anxiety I have ever had—not to mention the amount of medicine the doctors had me on. I knew things had to change, so I started weaning myself off what medicines I could. A friend found us a cheaper, smaller, quieter home in November 2015. Really a gorgeous place to heal that had only one floor, which is great for me. The cognitive issues, along with the blurred/double vision, make this home more suitable. I was finally approved for my disability benefits.

Friends have walked away, not able to handle *the new me*. The abundance of friends I have found with a similar injury as mine is amazing. They gave overwhelming support, and a listening ear, lots of understanding, along with words of hope and love from the TBI Tribe!

My life changed forever that day. As for the woman sitting next to me on the tree, it was my mother who passed in 2005. She came and covered me in a cloak of calmness and love. She was a God-loving woman who instilled her strength in me. One year to the day of the accident, I awoke to her next to me in bed. It was a vision, a very clear one. The woman at the tree was my beautiful Mother, keeping me safe like she always did when she was here. I am blessed.

The butterfly larva was gone and the lady "bug" was born! I was saved that day for a reason, regardless of the DAILY struggle. I awake to a new me every day! I have short-term memory loss, I fall a lot, have more pain then is bearable some days, plus vertigo and double/blurred vision. I sleep often, or not at all. This is an amazingly hard journey, and *I will not give up*! My new nickname is "Fifty First Kate's. They say laughter is the best medicine, and with the loss of memory, and not knowing what the next day will bring, I have embraced this nickname and have become proud to be called it by my friends.

What I want people to know and understand about a brain injury is that you must be very patient with yourself. Surround yourself with love and people who understand the journey. Leaving my other married life behind, and doing this on my own, has been one of the hardest things I have ever done—and also the most rewarding!

I will one day have a platform for women who put up with the mean words and actions. My husband may not have meant to crash that day, but no one deserves abuse or having someone in her life that doesn't have empathy and understanding, whether it be words or actions. I am here, I am strong, and I am not alone, and either are you. With hope anything is possible. Life is a journey not a destination. *Survivors and caregivers, stay strong because you are all amazing people.*

> I use to be a social butterfly, and that I cannot lie.
> On a hot summer day, in an instant she flew away.
> The reason I did not die, I may never know.
> Now I am a pesky housefly, who is often pushed away.
> I BELIEVE one day I will be a lady "bug" and make a wish come true.
> Fly to someone just like me, who hit her head so tragically.
> This journey is unknown, and most of the time we feel alone.
> Through tears, trial and time comes triumph.
> For I am only a lady "bug" who wants the world to know.
> We did not ask for this change in our lives.
> I am a lady and that will always be,
> Just remember I am also a "ladybug"
> And this one is going for advocacy!!
> – Kathy Duffy

No bio provided.

Chapter Forty-Seven
Seeing Brain Rages First Hand

Dr. Kevin Morford
Edmond, Oklahoma

My first experience with some of the bizarre aspects of the human brain came at the age of 21. I was a nursing assistant at a major hospital in Grand Rapids, Michigan, and one of my regular duties was acting as a "sitter" for people who were thought to be a threat to either themselves or others. The job was much like it sounds. My role was to make sure they didn't pull out IVs that were delivering important medicine, or yank out the catheters draining their bladders. Most of the time it was an uneventful, borderline boring day.

One spring day in early 2003 was anything but boring. I was assigned to sit with a man we'll call John. As I prepared to relieve the assistant who had been with John during the night, I got my customary report detailing some of the things I needed to know. Since John had come in late the night before, and had spent most of the time sleeping, there wasn't much to report. The only thing that stood out was a quick mention that he had suffered some degree of brain damage—we didn't yet know exactly where the damage had occurred or its severity—and he occasionally changed personalities.

Uncertain of what this meant, and with at least a little trepidation, I walked into the room. To my surprise, John was a cool guy. He invited me in warmly, thought it was fun I'd be spending the day with him, and even asked me what I wanted to watch on television. I thought I was in for one of the easiest days ever. No bedpans or sponge baths today. Eight blissful paid hours of TV and conversation were the visions swirling around my head.

Those visions didn't last long.

After barely an hour together, something strange happened. John suddenly, without any warning or indication he would do so, completely changed personalities. In a single heartbeat, he went from a guy who'd I like to be my friend to a belligerent, angry, threatening, foul-mouthed, raging lunatic. His face and body reflected the madness as he postured to fight while screaming a steady stream of four letter words at me. I stood there stunned, eyes the size of golf balls, doing my best to make sense of what was happening. Sure, my morning report had casually mentioned that he seemed to change personalities. It completely failed to mention that it happened so fast and to this degree. But it's also possible they didn't even know this yet. This behavior went on for what felt like an hour, but I think lasted less than two minutes.

Perhaps the most fascinating phenomenon is what came after. As quickly as John had fallen into a red-faced tirade, he calmed back down. The lights seemed to turn off and come back on like someone was flipping a light switch in his head. What was even stranger, he fully remembered his angry outburst laced with accusations and verbal abuse, and felt honest remorse for his actions. He apologized repeatedly, and you could see the agony consume his entire body as he began to realize *even he didn't know how to control himself.*

Most of our morning went through this repeated cycle. A kind, caring conversation of two guys hanging out, with a sudden interruption by rapid and total personality change with unbridled anger and profanity, was followed by apologies and confusion. It was like being in a room with the Incredible Hulk or Dr. Jekyll and Mr. Hyde. With each cycle I became wearier of John as I tired of the mental and emotional toll it took on me. But it was also painfully obvious that John was growing more tired, frustrated, scared, and weary of himself.

Which is why this eventually happened.

Shortly before lunchtime John's wife made it to the hospital and was cleared to see him. She had been given a brief report much like mine about her husband's condition, and how he was being affected. Today when I share this story with students and audiences, I always ask them to put themselves in her shoes. The person you love most dearly is in the hospital following a car accident. You're grateful they seem okay, no major physical injuries to speak of like broken bones or lacerated organs, but now you're being told that their personality unpredictably and wildly shifts from kind and caring to uncontrolled madness. Now imagine yourself walking into that hospital room.

At first the reunion was as sweet as you could script in the best romance movie. John and his wife embraced each other and shared repeated heart-warming affection saying, "I love you." His wife mentioned how happy she was he was okay, and John told her how happy he was to see her. He told her how confusing it was, and she tried her best to listen and understand. But again, putting yourself in her shoes, do you really think you could understand?

Of course, it didn't take long for one of John's outbursts. Now he had more ammunition than the one guy whose job it was to take the abuse. John laid into his wife as much as he did me. And once the outburst was over, John was crying with remorse and regret for treating her that way. You could already see how upset and confused she was. The man she knew and loved was different, in ways outside of what anyone yet understood.

It finally all came to a dramatic climax. With palpable tension filling the room like a heavy, dense fog, John completely lost his wits. In the middle of his raging and cursing, he threatened to throw his wife and me out the very real fourth story window in the room. Based on what we did know about how John's brain was working, it was clear this was not an empty threat. He could, and potentially would, try to follow through on this threat.

I immediately ushered his wife out of the room, and then went back to John. Moments later his rage subsided. But now he remembered threatening to kill his wife. As quickly as I can ever remember seeing someone in a hospital gown move, John was jumping out of bed and heading for the door to, as he put it, "go for a walk." He clearly meant, "I'm going after my wife."

Seeing where this is going, I get right beside John and start telling him that he can't leave, I can't let him go, and begging him to go back to his room. We're walking around the neurology floor in an escalating race where we are each trying to get a step ahead of the other. As we go faster and faster, almost to a run, we reach the big double doors that lead to the elevators. John takes off in a full sprint. Only my knowing his obvious intention, aided by the fact that I was wearing actual clothes and shoes, opposed to his bare feet and open-backed hospital gown, did I beat John to the doors and block his exit. But guess what happened.

John once again loses his composure. He's screaming, yelling, and cussing loudly for everyone to hear. His threats are flying in my face as he pushes and shoves to get past me. His heart is begging to apologize to his wife while this young kid (me) is annoyingly preventing him from doing just that. It's my highest obligation to not let him go. Can you imagine what might happen if someone in John's condition was let loose in a hospital with thousands of people milling around? I wanted to stay more of a barricade than a punching bag. I waited to get punched, but somehow he never hits me. And suddenly it's over.

Realizing he wasn't going to get through, John ran back to his room. I remember telling myself that I handled the whole situation very well. But when I went to open the door, my hand was trembling uncontrollably reaching for the doorknob. John had barricaded himself inside and wouldn't open the door. Doctors and nurses rushed to my aid and quickly decided that my presence was only going to make the situation worse beyond this point. I was promptly reassigned to another unit.

I don't know whatever happened to John. After that day I was never assigned to his care again. At that time we knew very little about the brain's ability to heal and recover. I hope that through all of our learning, John was able to find some healing for his damaged brain—and peace for his heart and mind.

Dr. Kevin Morford is a speaker, author, and chiropractic physician with a certificate in chiropractic neurology. He has 15 years of experience in the health and wellness industry. Dr. Morford also currently serves as faculty at Oklahoma State University in Oklahoma City while maintaining his private practice.

Chapter Forty-Eight
Broken-Hearted Mom

Kimilie Drew
Concord, New Hampshire

I'm the broken-hearted mom who has to advocate for my son until my last breath. Our family was devastated by a car accident on Mother's Day of 2015. My son was 16 then, and his coma lasted for almost two weeks. He received a severe traumatic brain injury, and the words still sting today.

From the very first day I was told by the doctor what we could expect if he recovered, I had to believe otherwise. I stayed by his side the entire time, as did many others from our family. He is a miracle and really the hardest-working young man who struggled to do the basic of tasks. So after we spent months in the hospital watching and helping him regain his life again, we go home from the rehabilitation program.

Because the driver had poor insurance, our son receives no wrap-around care. There is no follow up on anything by this state, and in fact, the state denied services for him because he was not injured enough!!!

I am outraged by the insult to injury he will endure the rest of his life because of a teen's bad driving choice. His life is a shell of the old one, even though he continues to work on just being.

I am angry that the life I had been looking forward to for him is no longer. I am at the same time grateful that he's with us, and I will continue to be his biggest supporter.

Kimilie is the forever-heartbroken mom/caregiver of the most courageous, determined TBI survivor, her now 18-year-old son. With the help of his sisters, Mom and Dad, Hunter is a miracle.

Chapter Forty-Nine
Dear Survivor

Krystal Decker
Windsor, Ontario, Canada

Dear Survivor,

You just survived a miraculous thing called a brain injury. You're scared. I get it. I was a teen survivor of a car accident. It happened right across from my house February 23, 2007.

You get headaches or migraines, you forget things, you're still a little clumsy on your feet, and you may have broken bones. It may take you a few months or maybe years to recover, or maybe you will be in recovery mode all the time, and that's okay. You will make adjustments to how you do things.

Don't give up on your dreams; simply change them to how you now live your life. It's hard, I know because I was 15, and once my body healed on the outside and I no longer had broken bones, swollen face or bruises, I didn't have friends, people pretended to be my friends, I never got invited to do things.

As you get older (if you were a teen when it happened), you will learn to just go with it. Don't give up on dreams. I had many dreams, or thought I wanted to do something, like be a sign language interpreter, and was told, "It'd be too hard." I took the classes that could help me, but when that career wasn't going to work, I modified what I wanted to do. I wasn't going to let anyone tell me a career in helping people wasn't going to work because I wasn't emotionally strong enough. No, I finally found something I could do when I took Community Service Worker

What I am saying is do what you love, and don't let anyone stop you.

Let's talk about being an advocate. Being a survivor you will need an advocate in your corner, whether it's your partner, children, or even your parent. It can be annoying when they want to help—but let them help you as much as they can, but they still need to let you be independent. Don't let people push you to things you're not ready for. The biggest thing I let someone tell me, and now I have to feel like a failure, is I can't work in the fast-food industry because I can't multi-task. So I never applied for those kinds of jobs because I was told I would probably fail.

By listening to what other people say you can and can't do, they are limiting you. I say go for it, try something, and if you really can't, you will know that you at least tried.

If it feels like I am jumping all over the place it's because I want to give survivors and caregivers as much possible within this story.
- When at doctor's office or any type of testing, be as accurate with describing symptoms of any kind. It does not matter how embarrassing it may be.
- Be as accurate as possible when describing a symptom, and don't downplay it, or let others downplay it, and say it's nothing.
- If you think it's important to tell your doctor, mention it.
- If you're seeing an occupational therapist, explain things that are happening.
- If you get mad at the tiniest thing, or burst in too tears for no reason, mention it.

I wish someone would have introduced me to the local brain injury support group in my area. It was a lonely world when none of the kids at school knew what I was going through.

Next let's talk about finding things you enjoy. Enjoy books? Great! Don't hesitate to join a book club or start one yourself. Ask your public library if they have multiple copies of a book, and just sit and talk for an hour or so. Maybe if it's a small town, you could do it at a different member's house each month. Find an activity and do it.

The best thing for recovery is to do things you enjoy doing so that you feel like yourself. Learn new skills, learn an instrument, try new recipes; whatever you do don't give up your passions. Be spontaneous in what you do. Don't do things you're going to regret. If you want to go to a big event, even if it's a graduation, prom or some reunion, go even if you don't have a date. What do you have to lose? Lastly I hope you have a great support system of family, friends, and professionals.

Krystal was involved in a car accident at the age of 15 on February 23, 2007 attempting to cross the street after a friend and her father dropped her off at home. She woke up the next day in a hospital in a different city. At age 25, she is a full-time volunteer.

Chapter Fifty
An Unexpected Four-Legged Friend From the Darkness

Kurt Trahan
Scott, Louisiana

Very few people know even some of my backstory, and only my wife, Heather, knows the true extent of how life has changed for me since that spring day in 2013. I hope that some of this can shed some light, possibly helping others who may be in a similar situation.

April 12, 2013 my family and I were heading towards Richard, Louisiana for an engaged encounter retreat. Heather was with me, pregnant at the time with our third child, and our two girls were in the back seat. We were about 5–10 minutes from the place on a small country highway. We came to a stop sign, and thinking it was clear, I pulled out. Unfortunately there was a truck coming that hit us while doing around 65 mph. We were all transported to the hospital, and were quickly released, thinking that everyone was okay. Only I was hurt, but none of my family.

To sum up the next 3-4 weeks, imagine the worst headaches that bring to your knees, plus confusion, dizziness, and nausea. After a few trips to the ER, I was referred to a neurologist. Another CT scan and MRI showed a brain condition that I have had from birth called Chiari Malformation. I had decompression surgery in August 2013 for this. It consisted of taking out a part of the back of my skull, opening the lining of my brain and cutting my first vertebrae to make room for my brain. All this was done a month before our son was born. I know that I have focused on spreading awareness of this in hopes of helping others, but I want to focus on the other side of what happened so that I am able to accept help and hopefully spread awareness.

When something traumatic happens, your body is programmed to react in a certain way to protect itself. In the case of the wreck we were in, I went into an abnormally heightened fight-or-flight mode because of the circumstances of having my family with me, where my life was at the time, and the severity of the accident.

I suffered a traumatic brain injury and concussion with post-concussion syndrome as a result of the car accident. Going through so much, between trying to recover from the wreck, and then the brain surgery, kept me in this heightened state. I was eventually diagnosed with post-traumatic stress disorder, which I refused to accept at first. PTSD was for the soldiers who went to war. I was just in a car wreck! I started noticing a change in myself from what I can remember. I say this because there are only sporadic periods that I remember for about a year and a half after the wreck. I don't remember so many of the little moments that I wish I could, much less the big ones, like finding out that Heather was having a boy, and when he was born.

The changes felt subtle to me, but not so much to those closest to me. The distance. The anger. The rage. The confusion. Then the blackouts. I wasn't the same person. I became a person that I didn't want to be around, and that was when I was able to realize what was going on. All the doctors were insistent that the blackouts were caused by something physical going on. All the tests that were run, all the blood work, all the studies came back negative. My diagnosis was a definitive *"This is an interesting case."* I really started to fall into the pit of depression, and it was beginning to envelop me with the hopelessness and the helplessness. And my brain was doing so much more, but I couldn't explain or figure it out. I had always heard about the loneliness and darkness that people talked about with depression, but *you never understand it until you are there.*

The deepest of the pit came to me two times; once I attribute to medicine I was on to hopefully treat the blackouts, and another to the PTSD. After the second one early in 2015, it was able to scare me enough to finally accept that I *was not in control anymore*. I needed help that those closest to me had been urging me to get, but I was convinced that I was stronger than whatever this was that I was fighting.

I finally went through about four months of therapy that turned out to be the best thing for me— but was also one of the hardest things I would ever have to endure. So many days I would leave the sessions so drained that all I wanted to do was go home to sleep, but I knew I had to carry on.

I had to realize in the sessions that the PTSD was my brain's response to the wreck, and my body had been in the heighten fight-or-flight response I mentioned earlier for over two years. Imagine a moment when you kick into fight or flight. It normally subsides pretty quickly. Now imagine living with that for two years. An absolute hell.

I then had to get my body to shut down this response. When it happened, all I could do was cry. And cry I did. I can't explain why. It seems like so many times in or after the sessions, all I wanted to do was cry. When your body is in a state like that, cortisol is stored which can affect so many things. After the response was turned off, and my cortisol levels came down, I dropped ten pounds in a matter of three weeks. It was such an amazing thing!

We were able to establish that the blackouts I had been experiencing were actually the physical manifestations of the PTSD. To explain it simply, with too much stress or triggers, my brain would shut down in order to cope. Now it was time to figure out how to manage these.

This is what brought the hard part. When the wreck happened, and my body went into the heightened state, it took in and stored all aspects that all of my senses were experiencing. These became my triggers. For instance, seeing the same color and style truck that hit us caused an instant anxiety attack. Hearing any type of scream, be it fear or arguing from my kids, triggered the instant of the wreck and hearing their screams then, was causing a flare up of symptoms. On bad days, I would have one of two recurring dreams—either reliving the whole wreck, to being in the hospital, or reliving it with the twist that everyone died. Sometimes I would have to relive this six to seven times a night.

I had to face these triggers and essentially reprogram them to be something good in my life instead of something associated with bad. This was much harder than I could have imagined, but with extensive help, I was able to get all of them down to a manageable level. Gone? No, but not affecting my life as much as before.

I do still have days, especially on the ones where the pain from the Chiari Malformation and corresponding brain surgery is really high, that the PTSD rears its head—and I see the glimpse of that person I don't like coming back. Even today, the old trigger of large groups came back when I attempted going to a gathering at church. Driving up I felt the tightness in my chest and started breathing like I had just run a 5k. My anxiety skyrocketed, but I tried pushing through so my kids could go have some fun. Eventually after a little while, I had to sit them down and explain that we had to go because Daddy's brain wasn't able to handle all the people right now.

A good friend of ours, who is in the military, mentioned PTSD service dogs. I had never thought of this route until that moment. I started doing research into these services and saw the hope of so many other people just like me who were helped by a dog trained to sense the PTSD attacks coming, and then calming the person. It was such an overwhelming ray of hope like I had not had in a long time. I was able to make contact with a couple of organizations that specialize in these services, and they look promising. I reached out to them, but was discouraged by the prices ranging from $10,000 to $20,000 for a trained dog, or that they only serve veterans.

So, not being the type of person to stop, I started doing more research into the Americans with Disabilities Act (ADA) and found out that I did not need to get a trained dog from a certified group, but rather I could do the training myself. Another ray of hope! I started a GoFundMe account for the original task of getting a trained dog, but only raised around $450. I happened to check the Craigslist posting for pets one day and noticed an ad for a nine-month-old Australian Shepherd. I contacted them right away, and was able to get the dog with all supplies and have enough money left over for training supplies.

The dog, named Obi Wan Kenobi, needless to say quickly became part of our family. He was originally purchased from a breeder in Missouri to be a PTSD service dog, and through a series of events, made his way to Louisiana. I started basic obedience training right away, but I noticed that he was keenly cued into me, especially when my anxiety was high. One night, for instance, I was watching TV by myself when a panic attack hit. Obi raised his head, ran over to me and put his front paws in my lap and started nudging me. Right away my anxiety tapered down.

A couple weeks later, I was having a rough day and went into a blackout. My wife and kids started doing the usual things of making sure I was laid out, comfortable and still breathing, but this time my wife let Obi out to see what he would do. He ran straight to me, jumped on my chest and started licking my face. I came out from the blackout within seconds, something doctors and modern medicine were not able to do. Absolutely amazing moment!

From there Obi's training and our life together continued as our relationship became stronger. He has helped me numerous times after the first incident. He still has his puppy and troublemaking dog moments, but who doesn't? Obi has become a regular around town and at church with me. People are genuinely curious about service dogs, but are hesitant to ask. On my good days, I try to make an effort to educate anyone who wants to know, but some days I just want to be in our little world and get home. I started a Facebook page for Obi in the hopes of spreading awareness and education, and as a way to continue helping me to live with and cope with my life as it is now. We have started doing some talks together, which has been great. This is a whole new path in our lives that we have to make the best of and use the new tools we are given. Easy? Hardly, but certainly worth it.

I am not telling all of this for sympathy, but rather in hopes of spreading understanding, and for anyone who might be going through this struggle.

To anyone who reads this, make the best of life, my friend.

Kurt is a husband to an amazing wife, Heather, father to three kids, and an engineer in the great state of Louisiana. He is a traumatic brain injury (TBI) survivor who works to provide support to other survivors through information, awareness and understanding. Outside of all this, he stays busy with camping, his service dog Obi Wan Kenobi, church activities and living life to the fullest.

Chapter Fifty-One
What I Can Remember

**Lee Staniland,
Ventura County, Oxnard, California**

It was June 11, 1978, in Somis, California, so I've been told, because you see, I have no memory of what happened that day. I know that I had just returned from Arizona where I became the godparent to my young nephew. My mother came back with me, and for Mother's Day, I had taken her to Solvang for the day. I also remember taking her to the Burbank Airport for her to go home.

Although I remember all that very clearly, I remember nothing from the actual day of the accident. Often I have been told different things so that they now have become my memories—like I had been outside washing windows when my husband left to go somewhere. I was probably upset about something or someone because that's when I'd wash windows.

I put my dogs up in their kennel like I always did when I rode my horse. My husband came home and could not find me anywhere until he looked out in the pasture located in front of our house. My then-husband told everybody that he had always told me not to ride when I was alone.

He noticed my horse with her bareback blanket on, and a hackamore hanging from her neck. He found me unconscious underneath one of the walnut trees in the pasture.

He gathered me up and took me to Camarillo's Emergency Room, and they transferred me immediately to Ventura's Community Hospital where I was in a coma for six weeks.

People have told me stories of things that happened there, like they left me in front of an open window one day, so I caught pneumonia as a result. Another time they kept giving me Dilantin to control seizures, and I was allergic to it. Because of that, I was scratching myself so badly that they tied my hands to the bed so I could not reach any part of my body.

They must have done most things right though, because I'm here today to tell you about it. When I came out of the coma six weeks later, I was sent up to Santa Barbara Rehab where I spent another 2 or 3 months.

Now about 18 months later, I had my first memory that stuck. I was in a room all by myself, and I could hear people out in the hall. I had no idea where I was or why I was there.

I have memories of little fragments of that time, like being with my family, my sister wheeling me around their hotel pool, another sister taking me for a car ride around Santa Barbara and lunch at Micky D's. Funny, the things you remember.

My husband took me out of the hospital to spend the day in Solvang for our first anniversary. That was a super memory. I got to be out of the hospital for a *whole day*. Wow!

I recall trying to walk down the hall with a walker, and not doing so well. One day to be funny, my brother hid the belt that the nurses had tied around me so I didn't fall out of the wheelchair every time I thought I could stand up on my own.

A great young gal was supposed to be with me while I cooked a meal I had chosen. No way I could do that yet, so she and her boyfriend cooked and ate a steak dinner—or whatever it was that I had picked out to try to cook. It was so much fun just watching them enjoy it. It still puts a smile on my face whenever I think of it.

Then there is the memory of crying and pleading with my family to take me home. They all felt so bad and wanted to do it, but they knew I wasn't ready, so they would leave and I would just fade out.

That is the good thing about not having a good memory. You forget most things that upset you. I remember things a lot better today, but at times, especially when I am tired, the old memory just doesn't work the way it used too.

Well, I finally got to go home, and I was so happy.

My parents had moved down from Sacramento to help take care of me. I had to relearn to walk, talk, dress, and feed myself. My old self was a very headstrong person, but I just let everyone help me with life. It's amazing how your mind protects you from yourself.

After awhile it was time for my parents to leave. I loved them so much but my parents were smothering me, and I wanted *my* house back. I know my mom was so afraid to leave me to handle things on my own, but it was the best thing for me.

Here's a secret for all you caregivers. Yes, it is a lot easier if you just do everything for us, but please don't. After my parents left, I had to do everything myself, from taking care of a big house, to caring for cows, chickens, dogs, cats and helping to run a carpet supply warehouse. I believe that is how I got to be as good as I am. I sold my horse because I could not ride her then. And I just remembered that my rooster would chase me whenever I would go out to collect eggs. They always go after the weakest thing—and that was me.

And, my husband and I were also still in the process of finishing the house we were building and living in. Talk about crazy!

I am so thankful that the part of my brain that reasons things out was not damaged completely. Don't get me wrong. I know that there are times when I get a little crazy about things. Maybe other people who do not have a brain injury would handle a situation a lot differently, but I do the best that I can.

I am now remarried to a man who does pretty well for someone who was not with me from the beginning of my brain injury. He has learned a lot from me, and I have learned a lot from him.

When someone says to me, "Oh, your head injury must not have been very serious," I would like to shake that person. I had to work very hard to get where I am. I had someone looking over me, and He decided that my time was not up yet, and I have something I'm still suppose to do. I believe my purpose in life is to be with my fellow brain injured, and to give them and their families hope.

Now almost forty years later, I am very satisfied with my life, and maybe that is because I have been given most of my old self back. And then maybe it is because I have some of the best people around me. So here is a Big Thank You to all those wonderful people that have stuck by me thru thick and thin.

I love you!

Lee's TBI was June 11, 1978. She now lives near the beach in Oxnard, California and is happily married to Buster Staniland for 21 years.

Chapter Fifty-Two
A Tumor the Size of a Walnut

Lisa Cohen
Mount Kisco, New York

I was twenty-three, living on my own and attending graduate school when doctors discovered a mass on my brain. Unaware of how a brain injury could affect someone, I was told not to worry, and to finish the semester. When I went to class the following week and couldn't focus, no longer could I go back to my studio apartment and pretend nothing changed.

One MRI altered everything; I moved back home, scheduled brain surgery, and hoped everything would be all right. I worried for days over how many pairs of socks I should pack for the hospital, and if yoga pants would be acceptable patient attire. Nobody told me none of that mattered. I was reassured brain surgery wasn't as scary as it sounded, and I would be fine.

May 20, 2014 I checked into the hospital in Connecticut for surgery. I walked along the hallway to the preparation room slowly following my nurse, until I realized *what I was walking towards*. For a while I stood there, staring down at my shoes… and cried.

When I woke in my bed seven hours later, my head was tightly wrapped in bandages, I couldn't move, or see, but I felt. I felt everything, and it was not fine. Through my eyes, the room was not a hospital room because I now had drastic double vision, which distorted everything. Because the tumor was on my cerebellum, removing it caused damage to my body. I couldn't tell who or what anything was, and I closed my eyes for most of nine days.

When a physical therapist tried to help me walk, we realized that because of the surgery, I now had ataxia/coordination problems on the entire left side of my body. I could not balance, use my left hand, or judge the distance between objects and walls. In the middle of one night, I tried to leave the bed on my own, but I couldn't walk, and slammed into a curtain and the wall. This prompted the staff to put a bell on my bed and a yellow star above my door, labeling me as a fall risk.

It's now two years later, and I have lived a very different life at an inpatient rehabilitation hospital with months of outpatient physical, occupational, speech, vestibular, and vision therapy. I never imagined that I would wake up every day struggling to walk, balance, read a book, or pick up a carton of milk.

I am now twenty-six and finishing my masters of fine arts in Creative Writing. Although I still (and may always) have ataxia and double vision, I went on to teach with a "right to write" prison program assisting women. I have found strength in helping others discover their voice, and also discover my own. I published my memoir about recovery and life since doctors found my tumor that was about the size of a walnut. Even though the tumor is now gone, my brain injury has become a part of me, and I'm okay with that—for the most part. I attend traumatic brain injury support groups, brain injury walks, and national brain tumor events where I aim to help raise awareness.

Although I still struggle at times, fall at train stations, and lose my voice, I realized I am here. I am here because no matter how weak my voice can be, it can be heard as I share my story.

Lisa at the age of 23 had brain surgery to remove a tumor from her cerebellum, which left her with double vision and ataxia. She is currently working on her MFA, training for a thru-hike of the Appalachian Trail in 2017 while advocating for brain injury support and awareness.
www.facebook.com/walnutmemoir

Chapter Fifty-Three
Living My New Life

Louisa Reid
Brisbane, Australia

When I was 56 years old in July 2013, I went to a computed tomography (CT) test to treat what I believed to be an earache. However, they found two aneurysms in my brain. My first one, to be operated on 293 days later, was 8mm, and the other was 5mm. Apparently the second one didn't need the same operation, and so it still lurks in my brain.

I did some research on Google, because I needed to know what was going on in my brain. I joined a support group on Facebook. On 22 April 2014, I went into surgery expecting that it would go well, and I'd stay in the hospital ward for a few days, and then come home.

In the intensive care unit (ICU) I couldn't really hear or understand when the ward staff spoke to my daughter about how I was doing. After one week I was shoved into a wheelchair and pushed across the hospital property to Brain Injury Rehabilitation Unit (BIRU), into the locked ward with staff, where my suitcase and me were unloaded onto my bed. I couldn't understand what was happening; it seemed serious, but I had no information. I cried and cried, and waited.

The next day I packed myself and went to the locked door to wait. No one wanted to let me out, so I stood in the hallway by the door. I went into the gym and waited in there, looking at the other door. I sat with my gear for quite a while. When an unsuspecting person opened the door, I made it out. I was stopped in the hall outside the locked door. I cried and refused to move back, and I refused to allow any staff to lead me into the locked area. It was like this the entire six plus weeks I was there.

A doctor rang my daughter, who arrived in an hour to talk to me. She calmly explained what was happening. She told me that I'd had a stroke with my operation, suffered a brain injury at my surgery, and had been taken to BIRU for support. I couldn't understand any of that, but I still had to turn back to the ward with the staff. I didn't want to stay on, but I had no choice. My daughter accompanied me back to my room.

The staff members who were supposed to support me would often be unable to help me as they helped so many patients with wheelchairs and bed chairs. There were far too many other BIRU clients who had ABI (acquired brain injury) or TBI (traumatic brain injury)—but I never included myself. Even so, I was frustrated because I didn't really feel I was moving ahead. I couldn't talk properly, I would repeat my own words, and realised that I wasn't replying in understandable words. I couldn't even use my laptop.

I was drawn into different training at BIRU. I had a speech pathologist, a music therapist, a physio, an OT instructor, and an instructor to walk with me. I was positive that I had turned my brain around, and I began to talk as if I could understand, even though I so often had to stop and think.

From the second weekend I was allowed to go home on the Friday afternoons, and return to BIRU on Sunday afternoons. I didn't, or couldn't, talk much. I stayed with my daughter only one weekend while another weekend I was with my dog sitters, and the rest I was on my own.

My daughter spent some special time with her spouse's mother, who was very sick with cancer, and she arrived back on the Monday morning. We had a full meeting with seven staff members to talk about my days. I had a "day end" of 6th June presented to me, and I had accepted it, but later the social worker told me that my day to leave the hospital was 18th June. I disagreed with any longer period, and agreed to continue to work toward the 6th of June.

My daughter picked me up on the Friday morning before she drove to the airport to fly out again, this time for her mother-in-law's funeral. After I got home I didn't feel relieved, but being home was necessary. My friends, who had stayed for more than seven weeks at my home watching my dogs, were due to move out on the 7th. I said goodbye to them—and was left on my own.

Whenever someone has brain aneurysm with or without a stroke, people need to understand how this thing is changing many lives. I read that 3–5 percent of strokes are caused by ruptured aneurysms. This doesn't include someone like me, with an unruptured aneurysm, which still lead to my stroke while in surgery.

Out of hospital I continued to attend speech pathologist classes for the next year, to work on what I still have: aphasia, a problem with my language. I also went to a Community Brain Injury Team (CBRT) where I worked with different people who would help me to recovery. Between my surgery and that time, I had been restricted from driving, and CBRT got me back driving after seven months.

I had joined a group on Facebook was a good for people with an aneurysm, and for so many other people who needed to find out information about aneurysms. I was taken on as an administrator, which I enjoyed. Most days for the last two years I posted information that probably many people would not know, and I felt it was safe to do this because of my language problems. For just over a year I also volunteered two mornings at a local art gallery. In 2015 I took a Stroke Foundation stroke management course, and later I took a Leader's course with STEPs (Skills To Enable People and communitieS).

Today I live in a "retirement" village. I know now that the result of the aneurysm and stroke is just part of my life. I have depression, which has hit bottom very recently, and I am working very hard to pull myself back up. For me, this is the result of living alone with no visitors. I'd lost most of my previous friends because of my TBI. Just before all this with the aneurysms happened, I had passed a Graduation Diploma of Occupational Health Safety, which complemented the job I'd had for seven years. Now I know I can't work in Workplace Health & Safety (WHS) because my brain won't remember everything I really should know.

Sometimes I feel very upset that I can't work anywhere. I have applied for jobs since my surgery, but most of them I never heard from; the ones who bothered to write said I didn't get their job. I can't make myself feel good because I keep thinking of what happened to me is as real as the cancer that killed my daughter's mother-in-law. Yet when I get up from the bottom of my depression I can think ahead, and I have gotten to know Acquired Brain Injury Outreach Service (ABIOS), Australia Aphasia Association, STEPs, National Stroke Foundation, Synapse and Brain Foundation—all Australian organisations that help people with stroke, and some which also work with brain aneurysms. I am also researching taking a course, which I think can help me get work.

I feel that many people are living some very difficult lives from having a ABI or TBI from aneurysms and strokes. I am determined to make more people aware of what a brain aneurysm and/or stroke can do to them or their spouse or friend.

Louisa has become very conscious of the problems in her brain after her brain aneurysm and stroke with aphasia back in 2013, and hopes to be able to make the public aware. She is a member of organisations in Australia that support brain injuries. She lives alone with her dog.

Chapter Fifty-Four
Invisible Injuries Can be the Hardest to Diagnose ... and to Heal

Lynn Julian
Boston, Massachusetts

Here are my two TBI stories, one occurred in 2006, and the second, 2013.

TBI #1: October 2006

I was known as Cookie Cutter Girl, 21st Century Pop Superhero. I packed "Girl Power Pop" with a punch on 500+ radio stations and 30+ CDs Internationally. "Rolling Stone" called me "Nashville's Version of Fiona Apple." (PopSuperhero.com)

I had started that night very excited as I was about to play a popular, 40-year-old club in a major city—but I ended in an ER in Boston. In 25 years performing on stages all over the U.S., I've never fallen. (I guess I should feel lucky?) Then I slipped on an untapped stage cord, fell backwards and bounced my head on the stage until I knocked myself unconscious.

After that stage accident, I was left disabled, in a wheelchair, due to undiagnosed TBI in the base of my brain.

The appointment with my primary care doctor was disappointing. He told me to follow the other doctors' orders. I decided to "doctor shop" for myself, and made an appointment with a voice doctor to see how this injury affected my neck and voice. It felt like I had a bone in my throat.

I also suffered from Ehlers Danlos Syndrome (EDS) and Fibromyalgia. I slowly, painfully, learned how to do many things over again, including walking, during the next 5-6 years. In 2012, I found a new passion to pursue and began acting in short films in Boston's Back Bay (BostonActress.org).

Often I tried to sing, but out came a raspy voice, and playing my guitar was too exhausting. I stayed home, depressed, cancelling many performances as well as networking events where I lost the opportunity to promote my singing. Thank God for my dog. On nights like this that look so cruel and unfair, he is my shining light of love. My dog licked away my endless flow of salty tears many a night. Little did I know, he was already training to be my service dog. Near the end of October, Stinker was now a genuine "service dog," preventing and interrupting my fits of anger, crying jags and panic attacks. I am so grateful for the unconditional love that four- pound bundle of joy brings to me every day. Then my doctor wrote a letter validating my dog's work.

A few days after my fall, I had intense pain and a severe allergic reaction, so it was back to the ER again tonight. My skin itched all over, and my throat was closing. Along with chronic pain, the ER prescribed even more allergy and pain medications for me to add to my ever-growing regime.

To add insult to my injuries, I was struggling financially as well physically. In a bizarre twist, this 40-year-old Boston club had dropped their liability insurance mere months before my show there. Yes, shockingly, this is legal. I also discovered, as a "work for hire," I was not protected by OSHA workplace safety laws, either. They cover employees and patrons, of which I was neither. Since I was only performing there one night, I was considered a "work for hire."

When the first ER bill arrived, for $2,500—I couldn't even look at it long enough to remember. I'm afraid I'll be forced to sue the club, or stay in debt forever. And the club has not returned any of our phone messages. I had 2 overnights at the ER. I have 6 doctors. PT 3x/wk. No work for months. I'm probably looking at $10,000 in medical bills alone. AND ...Now I'm an out of work. Who would hire a Superhero who's afraid of tripping on cords! No unemployment check for us self-employed people to pay our bills either. Local musicians in the "know" say I will definitely get blackballed if I sue.

Poor Doug was wonderful, working on 4-5 hours sleep and trying to take care of me and the house too because I'm useless.

I had horrible nightmares—and paranoia has found me, and my PTSD raged for the rest of the day. I felt trapped, depressed, self-absorbed and cowardly... a prisoner in my own bed. I can't even get out of bed for very long because I can't tolerate the intense pain.

What I lost in the first month:

I need to write it down, so I can focus on more positive things. You know how babies continuously discover new things they *can* do? Well, during the first months of recovery, TBI survivors feel like they continuously discover new things they CAN'T do.

- My band and gigs, plus ability to network—all present and future income from performing music and competitions, as well as selling my products at events. This includes my ability to sing, play my guitar, dance or perform—and to write music.

- My personal life, including social life, as I have *not* left house in two months, except for doctors, as well as my sex life with my fiancé because I am too sick and it's too painful.

- My patience with my fiancé, my dog and people because chronic pain makes you cranky.

- My overall health, and I wonder if these related to injuries or side effects of the medications I take because I cannot get through more than a few hours without medication.

- My ability to bathe, shower, put in my contacts, and do my hair and makeup without pain or fear of falling. Also, I can't get in and ride in a car without pain.

- My ability reach without pain—and this happens when I cook, make tea, eat, carry things like groceries and laundry, and this includes my purse and my musical instruments.

My service dog has become invaluable to my daily living. I cannot leave the house—or sleep through the night—without his help.

My TBI injury has especially affected my joy of living—my freedom to leave my house without pain and fear, thus I don't get to see my extended family, and my fiancé, Doug, lost his spot on the bed to my service dog. And, Doug has lost me as a companion in so many ways.

At the end of the first month, I had 500+ unanswered emails, which is why I was so stressed out and depressed.

I finally caught a break in January, thanks to my "doctor shopping." I found a facial surgeon who immediately diagnosed me as having a "fistula," or hole, deep in my ear canal. This can happen, when you hit your head hard enough, and the fluid leaked out the hole will result in similar symptoms to TBI, along with extreme vertigo. Inner ear fistulas are fixable with surgery. She was *only* able to diagnose me upon sight because she had worked with the NASA who pioneered surgical repair of ear fistulas! Upon referring me to a surgical colleague, he agreed to do exploratory ear surgery as a favor to her.

Five months later, the surgeon, who did NOT think he'd find any holes in my ear canal, found…two of them, "perilymph fistulas" in the deepest part of my ear canal! He found and repaired the holes, but…my pain and tinnitus got worse! Now with temporary hearing loss while I recover from the surgery, I'm training my service dog, with treats, to "alert" me when someone enters the room.

Finally in August, 10 months later, Doug emailed my family in Maine, who had not yet visited me in Boston since my stage accident. He wrote: Lynn is in the hospital and VERY ILL!!!! "She was in the emergency room for 2 days and now is in observation. All of her family should come down. She is suffering with great pain and needs as much support as she can get."

The ER doctors gave me a spinal tap, which resulted in a "rebound headache," the worst two- week migraine of my life! Doctors and nurses were NOT educated about this condition. With lost muscle mass and more weight, I was under a hundred pounds. This hospitalization left Doug and me with life-long emotional scars from their abuse and neglect, which also caused great fear.

My primary doctor didn't treat my bone infection, so I needed a new doctor. My surgeon finally took pity and prescribed me two months of high dose antibiotics. He also gave me the life-changing motivation to work harder and walk again. He said, "I know you are in pain. I believe you. I've watched you waste away in that wheelchair. BUT, if you stay in that chair much longer, you may LOSE your choice to get out of it…forever! Your muscles will be gone and your joints may freeze up. I KNOW it hurts…but you must *fight harder, fight through the pain* to walk again."

His words were the mixture of wisdom and fear that I needed to put a fire under my wheelchair-bound butt. I spent the rest of 2007-2009 going from wheelchair to walking again, even if it was still with a cane. I worked my way through every kind of therapy: physical; speech; occupational; ocular; mind-body, etc.

In the fall of 2009, I moved to Boston to be closer to all the major hospitals. There I saw a kind, caring neurologist, who diagnosed me with a brain injury. Finally, it all made sense: I had a mild traumatic brain injury (TBI).

From the end of 2011 through March 2013, I found a new passion to pursue, acting. I'd been on stages since I was five, spending my last years performing as a Pop Superhero. Acting was a natural transaction, so I began taking classes and acting in regional short films and commercials. TBI made it MUCH more challenging, as it does almost everything. The bright lights and tiny print on the scripts gave me migraines. The 12–16 hours days were exhausting and took me days to recover. Yet, it stimulated the part of my artist's brain that needed to be creative. I was nominated as "Best Actress" for a New England Actors Best of Award (NEABO), slowly earned a substantial acting resume, garnered good press, and built a new website, BostonActress.org. This artist was thrilled to be reinventing herself.

Little did I know, my TBI journey was far from over.

TBI #2: April 2013

Doug and I were spectators at the Boston Marathon finish line when it was attacked. Suddenly, athletes' dreams turned into nightmares none of us will ever forget. In shock, we were stunned …until my dog violently scratched my face to force me to move. We ran into the closest hotel, with me pressing my panicked, flailing dog into my chest with both arms, terrified I'd lose him forever. Some people were in shock, frozen in place, blocking our way to safety. Others were screaming. Some were throwing chairs out of the way. Others were pushing, shoving and trampling in fear. I became a drill sergeant, barking orders at frozen people blocking the door to "walk, walk, walk!" After herding people to the back of the room, I led them out the back door to safety. People who did not see the explosion wanted to go back outside again. I hope I convinced enough people to change their minds…to help who I could, when I could, how I could. The bombing left my service dog afraid of sudden or loud noises, such as a car door closing, which is too distracting to do his job well.

The next day I went to a Boston ER to get my head, ears, and back checked.

Still in shock and denial that a terrorist attack occurred two blocks from my apartment, my neighborhood was now labeled "Ground Zero" covered in police tape. Most mistakenly I believed my post-traumatic stress disorder (PTSD) came only from the bombing itself. However, I was equally traumatized, and re-traumatized, every day, over the following months, having to walk through "a war zone."

I spent the day after the marathon attack at the ER, hoping to get treatment for my low back pain, massive headache, slowed thinking, severe nausea, hearing "underwater," ringing in my ears, severe anxiety, and more. I angrily checked myself out, extremely disappointed, 7.5 hours later, receiving only an anxiety pill. The Boston ER doctors refused to treat my leg, ears or head, claiming there was nothing they could do. They told me to go to a doctor for my ears, my neurologist for my leg, and my counselor for my PTSD. The worst part was, on my medical release report, all they listed for my injuries was "anxiety." They did not even mention ANY of my other injuries…or any of my TBI symptoms. They specifically left out that a bomb exploded in front of me. I feared I would NOT be counted in the total "injured" by this attack. I wondered how many others with "invisible injuries," like TBI went undiagnosed—and possibly unaccounted.

Months later, in January I learned that my original TBI was to the base of my brain, which controls motor function. My new TBI was to my frontal lobe, which controls cognitive function. The year after the terrorist attack, a fellow survivor, also with TBI, told me I should see his physiatrist, which I did. He signed me up for vestibular therapy, to work on my balance. It takes one to know one. I noted TBI symptoms in several other survivors, encouraging them to seek evaluation. Each one did have an undiagnosed mild TBI and is now in treatment. (NOTE: Many with brain injury hate the label "mild." *No TBI* ever feels "mild.")

I felt like a "victim," rather than a "survivor," and needed to do "something" to feel more in control and empowered. So, I trained every day, for five months to run the 2014 Boston Marathon. I completed that race, in the Mobility Impaired division, along with the Boston Athletic Association's (BAA) Half Marathon, 10K and 5K races, collectively called their "Distance Medley." I am so honored to be named one of the "Most Inspirational Women to Ever Run The Boston Marathon" by "SELF Magazine." (see link below)

In the Summer 2015, I auditioned for my first film since my second TBI, "Witch Hunt," and was cast as the Evil Nun in this Indie Horror movie. I was also relieved my parts could be filmed all in one day because people with TBI need extra breaks, more rest and lots of sleep.

In 2016, I had noticeable TBI improvement from HBOT treatments, which reduces my PTSD by half, and increased my cognitive ability. I also started using CBD oil to successfully prevent and interrupt my panic attacks, which also reduced my inflammation and chronic pain.

Lessons I've Learned:

- What I now know, ten years post TBI, is that there is *nothing* I "can't do." I simply have to figure out how to do it differently that before my TBI. I must continually adapt!

- YOU are your own best advocate. Only *you* know what symptoms are "new" and what symptoms are "normal" for you. The foundation of your medical team is your primary doctor, so be sure to have one who will fight with and for you for your medical rights. Keep fighting for treatment of new symptoms, and don't stop until you are fully diagnosed!

- I did *not* receive a CAT scan or MRI at the ER. If you think you've got a head injury, *always* demand a brain scan!

- Your primary care physician is not a TBI specialist. I should have seen a neurologist immediately.

- Try to take only one new medication at a time. This allows you to see how you react to it and what side effects you have from it.

- Your brain needs REST! It is critical that you limit access to computer and phone screens, as well as reading for two months.

- Get a mini voice recorder, or set up alerts on your phone, to help you remember all these appointments and pills in a medicated fog!

I chose to do volunteer work because it gave my life purpose again. I chose advocacy because it gave me my voice back, not to sing, but to speak for those who cannot. The lesson is to find what speaks to you, and channel what energy you have towards it. Only you can decide what gives your life "purpose" and will make you feel good about yourself again.

My message is one of INSPIRATION and HOPE. I fought my way out of that wheelchair, and I fought my way across that finish line. If I can do it, so can you. Never give up HOPE!

Strength Through Unity…

Lynn Julian Crisci wears more hats than a Hydra has heads. In film, she's an actress in dozens of movies. In music, she's a Pop Superhero on 30+ CDs Internationally. In tech, she's a website SEO guru and a press release and article marketing writer. In health, she's an "Activist, Ambassador, Speaker, Consultant." Her daily struggle with chronic pain inspired her to volunteer as the Director of Medical Marijuana Advocacy for Leaftopia, which includes overseeing all their social media and fighting for patients' rights. She is the Massachusetts Ambassador for the US Pain Foundation (USPainFoundation.org), and the Advisory Panel of the Massachusetts Resiliency Center (MAResiliencyCenter.org). Her message is one of Inspiration and Hope.

www.Facebook.com/BostonFilm
www.Twitter.com/PopSuperhero
www.Instagram.com/BostonActress

Chapter Fifty-Five
From Victim to Survivor

Makenzie Biggs
Edmond, Oklahoma

December 12, 2007 was just like any other day in Edmond, Oklahoma. I was the typical freshman teenage girl, and at age 15, I was about to learn to drive. It was the first day back to school after a couple of days off due to an ice storm. My best friend and I lived in the same neighborhood so after school if I didn't have softball practice, we would always hang out together. On this particular day it was like all of the other days. We rode the bus home from school together. We went to her house and had our afternoon snack like we always did, and we hung out there until her mom got home.

I then grabbed my backpack and started to walk home. About halfway home her mom pulled up beside me in her white SUV containing my friend and her two little brothers. The mom rolled down the window and asked me if I wanted a ride home. I thanked her and said that I was almost home, so she said, "Step up on the car's running board so you don't have to walk." I was a very shy and timid, so riding on the side of a moving vehicle is something I would never do. Not to mention my mother is very strict, so she would kill me if the thought of riding on a moving vehicle even crossed my mind. I told the mom that I did not feel comfortable riding on the side of her car, but she was very persistent and insisted that I should not be walking home.

As I stepped up on the side of her car, I knew I was doing something wrong, but I kept telling myself it was okay because the mom told me to, and if a grown up tells a 15-year-old, it must be okay. As I'm hanging on to the side of the SUV, I feel the vehicle start to go faster and faster. Suddenly I feel my feet start to slip and then, all I hear is screaming.

I fell off the side of the SUV and hit my head so hard it caused me to seizure. I was lying on the ground completely knocked out. The mom called 911, and told paramedics that I was walking home from school and had a seizure and fell to the ground. I had no outside trauma, so the paramedics didn't know she was lying. She failed to mention anything about me hitting my head, so paramedics had no clue that my brain was bleeding. Since paramedics were given false information about my conditions, they did not provide a backboard or neck brace. They were on the scene with me for over 20 minutes.

However, with brain trauma, patients have to be at the hospital *within 20 minutes* after paramedics arrive at the scene.

Finally after four hours at the hospital, I still wasn't responding, so the doctors started to question things and took me in for a CT scan. The doctor came rushing back to my mom and asked, "What the heck happened to her? She has a skull fracture and a large blood clot on the right side of her brain." He left to talk to my friend's mother on the phone. He came back and told my mom that I fell off the running board of a SUV. My mom was shocked because like I said, that is something I would have never done. I was in the ICU for four days and in the hospital for a total of a week. The doctors told me that I was borderline, and was the closest case they've seen that has turned around and ended up not needing to have brain surgery.

Doctors do not prepare TBI survivors or their caregivers for what is about to come. No one tells you that the next several months are going to be hell. I had no idea what was about to come my way—that I was going to have horrible migraines every single day. No one explained to me that my mind would be that of a 6-year-old, but to me I would think I was completely normal. I had no idea why I was always so tired or got so frustrated over the littlest things. No one explained to me that the minute I left the hospital, not only would my life change, but also my mom's life. It took us many months to learn what to expect from *the new me*.

My mom was a single mom. My two brothers are seven and five years older than me, so for the last several years, it had just been my mom and I. The accident was a couple of weeks before Christmas break, and I did not return to school the rest of that semester. I started physical, occupational therapy and speech therapy. Doctors told me that I would not go back to school all year—and that I would not be driving by the time I was 16.

God made me hardheaded and strong-willed from day one. If someone tells me that I can't do something, I want to prove him wrong, so that finally worked to my benefit in this situation. I proved everyone wrong. Starting that January I returned to school one class at a time. I couldn't handle going to all my classes because I would get too overwhelmed and too tired. Slowly but surely I was able to go to school for half a day. By the time I was 16, I was driving. I got my license a few months late, but nonetheless I was still driving when I was 16.

I continued to beat the odds—everything that the doctors told me I couldn't do—I did. I remember when I was going to speech therapy to work on memory techniques, my mom was talking to the therapist about college. The therapist told my mom not to worry about college because she needed to focus on getting me through high school right now, because I'm not like my brothers, and I shouldn't be thinking about college. In other words she didn't think I was capable of going to college.

I applied at Oklahoma Christian University and was accepted. One of my doctors told me I had no business taking more than 6 credit hours at a time, and it was not about how long it takes me to graduate, but about whether or not I even graduated. My college adviser, my mom and I sat down and discussed my classes for first semester. After a lot of talk, my advisor finally convinced my mom to go against doctors' advise and let me take 12 credit hours. She explained to my mom that I had an easy load, and I would be a part of OC bridge program, which was designed to help students who needed any assistance throughout college. Honestly, if it weren't for the bridge program, I wouldn't have made it through college. They helped me transition from high school to college. I started by taking 12 hours, and by the time I was a junior in college, I was taking 15 hours. I graduated Oklahoma Christian University after five years, with a degree in family studies and child development, and a minor in education.

The hardest part of having a brain injury in college was trying to be the "normal" college kid, and still function. It was physically impossible for me to stay up till 2 or 3 a.m. and go to class like some of my friends would do. I would have killer migraines because my brain requires more sleep than most. About halfway through college, I finally faced the fact that I didn't care what people thought about me, like I can't handle being in big crowds because it makes me over stimulated. I'd have to leave, but I needed to do what's best for me.

It's been almost 8 years, and I've finally learned that I'm not "special needs" because I have a TBI. My accident does not define who I am, and I cannot be afraid to share my story. It wasn't until I was sitting at the doctor's office just a couple of months ago complaining about my headaches, when I truly realized how lucky I was. I asked the doctor how his patients with TBIs like me were doing with their migraines this many years out, and his exact words were "You don't understand, people with that type of injury don't typically survive."

Makenzie Biggs is a TBI survivor. She lives in Edmond, Oklahoma, where she currently works with developmentally disabled adults.

Chapter Fifty-Six
The Unfortunate Slip

Mary Frasier
Rice Lake, Minnesota

Yes, that unfortunate slip changed my life.

I had driven to work in a blizzard that February 26, 2009. My intuition kept hounding me to stay home. I had an hour drive from western Wisconsin to Minnesota where I worked in mental health with homeless women and children. The snow was heavy, the roads slippery, and it was coming down quickly. In hindsight, listening to that inner voice and staying home that day would have kept me on my journey towards the course of my dreams.

I started my day visiting clients, attending to their struggles, and feeling a sense of accomplishment as the day moved forward. I left a client's home before noon, hungry and ready to tackle issues. I recall walking around the corner—and then I woke up, lying in the snow, wondering where I was, and why I was in the snow. It took me a bit before I started to recall the day.

I had slipped on some ice, hidden by the mounds of snow. The files I had held in my arms were strewn all about. I didn't know what had happened because I passed out for a while. I think the cold snow helped revive me. I only knew that I fell because of the pain in my head. Prior to the fall, I'd been hungry. Now, I was shaking like a leaf, nausea set in, and things looked visibly foggy. Frightened, I called my supervisor, saying that I needed to go home, but she advised me to go to the doctor.

After driving an hour home in a blizzard, feeling weird and with a headache from hell, I made it to the doctor. A CT scan was done, a bump was detected, but no bleed, so all is well, and home I went to rest. Sleep was all I wanted at that point. I felt I'd be back to work the next day for sure.

Sad to say, it's been 7.5 years since that day, and I still have not returned to work.

It is a long, humble, strange, and painful physical and mental journey, filled with the sadness of loss. I had visual problems, memory, balance, vestibular, a labrynith concussion, nygstamus, aphasia, fatigue, and the most heightened sensory overloads that cause isolation. The neurologist explained that I had a labrynith concusion after the fall. This entails vestibular problems, which is damage to the inner ear nerve, causing balance problems. I had wondered why things looked foggy. I was told I had a nygstamus. A "what" I thought. A nygstamus is irregular eye movement, where focusing is difficult. This led to the inability to drive for months, and a huge lack of appetite. Another major symptom with the nygstamus and vestibular injury is fatigue, and headaches that turn into migraines for days. Then the sensory overload comes into play, with heightened noise, lights, and smells. The difficulties are endless.

The roller coaster of emotions is another challenge due to the multitude of losses. My job, home, income, outings with friends, family changes, and the most difficult navigation of Workmen's Comp, insurance, and disability hearings—all with a brain injury.

We are warriors in this most unexpected challenge. You have to be, or the consequences are great of falling into a deep depression. Many of us look and sound okay (until the sensory overload hits), which is why TBI is so difficult. Judgments about us run amuck all around us. We get it. We didn't even see some of our own deficits until years had passed. Those who are close to us, like my four beautiful adult children, can see those changes. My kids have been my eyes, ears, and comfort after the TBI. I'd had many knocks to my head as a kid from parental abuse, and thus I recognized symptoms I had struggled with after a head injury as a child. The struggles in speaking, writing, and attention were always present. We must be aware that children may have a TBI if maltreated. Then I had the one car accident in 2005, which added insult to the injury of the fall. So, recovery was tough.

We all learned to accept my change from a busy person to a tired, spacey, isolated person with numerous challenges. In time, we developed a healthy sense of humor about my random, inappropriate comments made without a filter. I drop things constantly; oh, my poor downstairs neighbor.

The TBI support groups have helped more than I can say with sharing similar experiences and being a place of great acceptance.

Boredom does not enter my life due to the constant need to find things I misplace, learning to create hobbies like crochet, knitting, finding lost things, bead work, finding lost things—yes, that takes up 35 percent of my day.

Meditation is so helpful, especially if using a guided CD or phone app. Even shopping for a short period of time, when not a lot of people are around, is still difficult because the sensory input of voices is louder than in the past. When I am at a restaurant, with noise and too many conversations to make sense of, you can be guaranteed I will say something that's weird, or leave with a migraine. We all want to be with others, so we push through moments, only to go home completely exhausted. Then we need lights off, TV off, and a comfy bed and pillow to recover. It can literally wipe us out for days.

I was pleased to speak on a survivors' panel at the Brain Injury Conference in Wisconsin one year. The need for education is greatly needed for doctors of all sorts, families, and ourselves, the survivors. Speaking at the conference with providers who care for patients helped them grasp a better understanding of TBI and the care they give to TBI patients. Doing this gave me purpose, and felt so good to give something to the TBI community.

I could say so much more as the challenges of the past 7.5 years have been unthinkable, uplifting, and humbling, but have also given understanding, and touched my soul in numerous ways.

This is a brief description of my journey and my hopes are it helps someone understand TBI a bit more. Many blessings sent your way.

Mary grew up in Rhinelander, Wisconsin and graduated in 1974. She has four amazing, beautiful, adult children whom she cherishes. Her interest and education were in mental heath and journalism, and she attended the University of Stout in Menomonie, Wisconsin. Prior to her education, she worked with battered women as a county advocate, training advocates and maintaining the care for the program. Two others and Mary started a runaway program in eastern Wisconsin around the same time. After her education she worked as a counselor at a Native American tribe, then as a supervisor overseeing a number of group homes for SPM (seriously persistently mentally impaired) adults in Wisconsin. Preceding those positions, she worked with SED (serious emotional disability) children for 9.5 years in Minnesota. And lastly, when the fall happened, with homeless, chemically dependent women with children. Mary misses the work so much! It was a long grieving process to accept the fact work was not an option after the brain injury.

Chapter Fifty-Seven
Body Painting: A Caged Mind

**May Mutter,
Ottawa, Ontario, Canada**

It all started in February 2013. I slipped on the ice while curling, hitting my head on a rock. I laughed it off, and carried on. Two weeks later while playing volleyball, I got hit directly between the eyes, which knocked me out before my head hit the floor. When I got up, I was still dizzy and couldn't see straight. I know now I should have sat down and given myself a chance to recover; it could've made all the difference.

I looked at this way: you don't run to the doctor every time you hurt yourself, yeah it hurts, but you suck it up and keep going. So I ignored the pain. The following week, I continued to play volleyball out of stubbornness, and this further aggravated my brain, and just the movement of diving around the gym floor, subjected it to yet another concussion. Like with a bruise—you don't keep poking at it to see if it's healed because that slows down the actual recovery process, but since everything we do is constantly poking at our bruised brain, no wonder it wouldn't heal.

The next day, I remember sitting at work with a bag of ice on my head and a cold bottle of wine in my hand to numb the pain. Eventually my coworkers forced me to go to the ER, where I was dismissed almost instantly. They gave me painkillers and told me I'd be fine in a week or two. I wasn't. I spent the first month and a half in complete darkness, and couldn't even carry on a conversation with my husband.

It wasn't until late May of that year that a story hit the news: a local high school girl died from getting a second concussion after ignoring her first. Only then did my doctors decide to actually start paying attention to me, send me for an MRI, and they also referred me to a concussion specialist.

I couldn't do my job and realized I couldn't even find new work that would accommodate my new situation. Insurance eventually agreed to short-term disability, but refused for almost three years to finally pay for long-term—I'm lucky that's changed because I had an amazing team behind me that encouraged me to get a lawyer involved and fight. To the insurance company, a board of doctors on the other side of the country claimed head injuries are a problem for a maximum of three months, after which you should be back on your feet. They requested letters from all of my doctors and therapists, but then stated it was "just an opinion," and continued to refuse my appeals.

Between that and no one being aware of my invisible injuries, I felt so alone. I'm considered a high-functioning survivor, yet getting through the day is constantly a challenge, which you would never know by just looking at me; so much of it is an act. The headaches, lack of concentration and focus, the light and noise sensitivities, my mood, and irritability level all spiked. To this day, only those close to me understand what I'm going through, and this is because I finally hit a point where I considered ending my life—me, the so-optimistic-you-can-call-me-naive person.

I felt so alone…so caged. All these things I wanted to do but couldn't because of my concussions.

I starting drawing and was asked to draw how the concussions affected my life: caged in a prison that happened to be my head. So I drew a picture of me with a bandaged head behind bars to make the invisible visible. Then I wrote a blog post about what went through my mind, and the number of people who've reached out to thank me was unbelievable. So many people felt so alone and so trapped, and they said that I put into words what they haven't been able to, which allowed them to share with their significant others and to even understand it themselves. So I started focusing on my message, "You are not alone," and thus, "A Caged Mind" was born.

Most information about TBIs is overwhelming and requires more reading than our injured brains can handle. So if I, the high-functioning survivor that I am, couldn't handle it, how is everyone else dealing with it? So I've decided to combine my previous life where I was a body painter, and my current broken one, to create A Caged Mind. I am currently body-painting people impacted by concussions to give a visual story of what a concussion is and how it affects us. It's about the symptoms, what to do, and what really goes through our minds, brought to life for people without TBIs to be able to visualize and understand, but also for people with a TBI to know they're not alone. I'm working on publishing this as a beautiful coffee table book that people would be proud to have in their homes; it serves as a purpose to spread the word and raise awareness about concussions as well as reach out to concussion survivors so they know they're not alone.

If only I had known to take it easy after my first hit, I may not have become disabled for life.

May sustained four consecutive concussions within three weeks in sports. With the belief that the invisible injury is an isolating journey, she is an advocate for brain injury awareness one body painting at a time. For more information on her project, A Caged Mind, check out www.facebook.com/thecagedmind and her blog at www.caged-mind.com

Chapter Fifty-Eight
Our Post-TBI Honeymoon

Melissa Jirovec
Cumberland Beach, Ontario, Canada

My husband and I had always dreamed of going to Australia. When we were in college, we'd considered continuing our education abroad, and spending a couple of years exploring the country.

My husband was in an ATV/dirt bike head-on collision that resulted in his TBI. After his traumatic brain injury in 2014, I decided that it was more important than ever to make our dreams come true. And so we planned our Australian honeymoon when he was well enough to make the trip. It certainly wasn't easy. Picture me, a 23-year-old newlywed pushing my husband in his wheelchair, while simultaneously pulling his walker and our luggage around several airports that spanned our 22-hour trip. I'm pretty sure I was functioning primarily on adrenaline at that point, but our excitement of what was to come kept me pushing forward.

When we arrived, we soaked up every detail of our surroundings: sounds, accents, language, and culture. We hadn't really made too many plans ahead of time so we could pick and choose our activities, based on my husband's fatigue levels. I'd like to start off by saying that our trip was incredible. We had our very own Australian adventure as a newly married couple, and for the most part, the trip was exciting, intriguing and a whole lot of fun. However, having not even hit the one-year post-TBI mark, there were challenges to our travel, as you can imagine. Fatigue and accessibility were two of the biggest obstacles, along with transportation.

At this time, my husband was able to walk short distances with his walker, and for longer distances he needed his wheelchair. By suppertime he usually was too tired to walk, so we used the wheelchair. Our first four days were spent in Sydney, and we were disappointed to learn that the taxi drivers there did not want to take us anywhere because of my husband's wheelchair. I didn't understand why because it folded up very well, and my husband had no problem going from chair to seat. But we were often met with dirty looks and given excuses as to why we couldn't be taken to our destination.

One particular evening, as we were leaving our hotel, we informed the hotel staff of our difficulties getting around. The concierge called us a taxi and put the wheelchair into the back of the cab before the driver had a chance to protest, then wished us a nice dinner. I could tell right away the driver was not happy about this, but didn't pay much attention to it. When we arrived at the restaurant, the driver proceeded to take my husband's wheelchair out of the trunk and throw it at me in the street. He then got back into his cab, and glared at me as I tried to set it back up with the cushions, while I was in the middle of the street, shaking, in a dress and heels. My husband watched helplessly from the cab, unable to exit until his chair was available.

I'm not sure my husband was fully aware of what had occurred, to be honest. I've never faced such cruelty from another human being. And for what? Because my husband was disabled? Because we weren't like everyone else? What had we done to deserve that? When I finally got the chair together, I quickly wiped my tears and helped my husband into it. The driver sped off, and I did my best to shake off the anxiety and hurt so we could have a nice dinner. We picked quite the spot for our dinner that night; a restaurant high up with a gorgeous view of the city and delicious food. I focused on the food and the beautiful scenery, and enjoyed a wonderful dinner with my husband.

Despite his mobility impairments, speech impairment, and cognitive impairments, we overcame the obstacles that we faced and enjoyed the trip of a lifetime. After almost losing my husband, I am eternally grateful to have had such a great opportunity, even if it had some fairly difficult moments.

Melissa Jirovec is a full-time caregiver, (non-practicing) registered nurse, an author and a certified Master Coach Practitioner hoping to work with caregivers of family members with acquired brain injury. She runs a blog on her website about her experiences as a caregiver and has spoken at several events about caregiving challenges and brain injury. At the moment, Melissa and her husband are enjoying their new role as parents to a sweet baby girl. www.melissajirovec.ca

Chapter Fifty-Nine
Not By Accident

Michael Ray Music
Burleson, Texas

In 1991, at 18-years-old, when my life as independent adult was just dawning, I was involved in a near-fatal accident, I had caught a ride with some college dorm friends back home for a weekend, and we were returning to school when life stopped. My reality and dreams would be abruptly altered without my consent.

We had just entered the freeway in the right lane when a semi-truck hit us while changing lanes. This caused us to run off the road into a ravine, and hit a tree at 65 miles an hour. Unfortunately, I was lying in the back seat with the top of my head facing the passenger side where the car hit the immovable tree. Also, unfortunately, the car was a Yugo, the late-eighties version of today's smart car.

An ambulance driver from that night later revealed that I was trapped in the car for almost thirty minutes before they could get the jaws-of-life to disentangle me from the wreckage. I was not breathing when they arrived. Fortunately, they were finally able to resuscitate me there, but then I slipped into a coma.

While I was in that comatose state, my parents were updated on my sustained injuries. I had broken my left upper arm, to the point that the bone needed a plate to seal it back together. Next, I had broken my right thighbone, and had to have a rod inserted to it to give it stability and strength to heal. I had also broken my right collarbone and my right shoulder blade, along with a broken rib.

But, incredibly that was not the worst injury. I had incurred a basal skull fracture, from the back of the head to the right ear, and I had sustained a cut on the right backside of my head. This all lead to the primary concern for the doctors: a traumatic brain injury.

While I was in the coma, my parents were told about this head injury. As the discussions with the doctors progressed through my two-and-a-half week comatose state, my parents were advised that because of the location of the area the brain that was injured—even if I were to come out of coma, I would need to be institutionalized.

When I did finally come to consciousness from the Glasgow scale 3 coma, I awoke to a new life, a paralyzed life. Through a haze of someone in a white coat talking to me about the injuries I had suffered, I remember sitting in my sterile hospital bed. I looked at myself for the first time in a mirror, in shock, at the visible evidence of the brain injury. The right side of my face drooped down severely, and I was not able to physically move at all. I was told the paralysis had to do with damage to the brain, and they were not sure how long it would last.

I began my rehabilitation in earnest, with various types of therapists: occupational, speech, and physical. I had to learn how to write, speak, and think again. Initially, I was having a problem picking out shapes and colors, and my handwriting looked like that of a preschooler. I was out of the hospital in two-and-a-half months, in a leg brace, and I was in outpatient rehabilitation for another four-and-a-half months.

A major obstacle from my TBI that has been hard to overcome is my moods. The therapists explained to me that emotional regulators in the brain had been eliminated. So, now, when I get angry, I go immediately to being furious, and when I am sad, I fall into depression. I have no emotional middle ground. Fortunately, in recent years I have been prescribed medication to help slow down my emotional reaction time.

Another challenge has been my short-term memory. I forget everything, and nothing seems to stick very long in my short-term memory storage. I've come to hate when people remark to me, "Hey Mike, remember when…?" Do you know who you are talking to?

Finally, I also struggle with feeling claustrophobic in my own brain. I have this thing that when too many things come at me, or are told to me, I began feeling overwhelmed. This usually triggers the emotional mood swing so I become angry. This became progressively evident when I began working jobs that required multi-tasking, which frequently caused me troubles.

All the above obstacles became very obvious and revealing when I married my wife in 1997. Suddenly, I was living with someone 24/7. Before, I could take a break from friends or roommates, but when I became a husband, there was no hiding. Even worse, I didn't know I even had a problem with these things. I knew I had initial problems in the hospital with my anger, which I had been warned about, but years had gone by as a single man, to the point where I didn't think I had any more problems. Little did I know—until my wife put that gold ring on my finger.

I would like those who read my story to gain hope, and not feel isolated any more. Hope, in the fact that the accident happened 25 years ago, and I am still here. I have been married for 19 years, and I have four incredible children. I have attained a Masters degree, but I still do struggle with the effects of the TBI, and continue to take medication. I also have to wear glasses, because my eyes demanded it. It's just one of those things.

I also understand that, as someone whose life has been altered by damage to areas of the brain, you can feel alone. Everyone around you is normal, but you are different. Something unalterable has happened to you, and because it is an "invisible injury," no one else understands your loneliness.

Only recently I have become aware of websites dedicated to TBI. Before I never understood that TBI was an actual thing, and it has been so refreshing and encouraging to become aware of other survivors of brain injuries. When you think you are alone, in your permanent injury, it definitely becomes harder to deal with.

My fellow TBI brethren, you can keep going. Search for something bigger than your injury, instead of just focusing on your limitations. I spent too many years focused on the cant's, and not pushing myself to think outside of the box—the box of your or others' expectations of you. If you keep looking back, you will never move forward. It is only now, at age 44 that *I am looking forward*. What can I do, and what am I good at? Don't keep trying things that are not working, but try something different that would work. Keep trying until you do find something that feels right, but maybe not the usual.

Then, find someone to help you get there, by planning and thinking outside the box. It is a great help to have someone who cares enough to believe in you. Personally, I have had *a lot of someones*. I have had mentors and friends to listen to me rant, question, and cry. I've had family to support me physically and emotionally. And I have had a wife to care enough to understand me and put up with me.

Most of all, I have had Someone to pray to, and ask help from, Who has given me the drive to push on, even when I didn't want to, sends me a friend when I needed one, and bring me a smile from a stranger. I received donations from churches during my family's time of need. He also blessed me with a wife when I thought no one would ever love me in my condition.

My fellow TBI brethren, please push on. Do not live by your limitations, live by the things you haven't tried yet. And most of all, find someones, a someone, and the Someone to lift you up and give you hope.

Finally, above all, whatever caused your TBI was not necessarily an accident. I believe everything happens for a reason, but Lord knows, I don't always agree with or understand those reasons. Even with the many problems and frustrations that have been caused by my accident, many great things have come from it.

The people I've met because of my delayed timeline, I never would have met. I have made some of the greatest friendships and relationships because of my detoured timeline. I would have never met the most perfect friend and wife if I hadn't had my life interrupted by a car accident in a Yugo, at 18. I've started saying that I would not like to live through the accident again, but I wouldn't change it.

Originally from Visalia, California, Michael now lives with his family—his wife of 19 years and four kids, in Burleson, Texas.

Chapter Sixty
"No Boundaries" Anymore

Molly Raymond
Fairfax Station, Virginia

I was driving home on a beautiful summer Saturday evening on July 2004. Just down the road, two cars were drag racing, and coming up on me quickly. Suddenly, I was struck in the rear by both cars, one hitting right after the other, causing my car to spin around violently and crash into a guardrail. That is what I have been told. I was knocked unconscious and remember nothing of the accident. The two cars that hit me were filled with eight high school students going 95 mph on a road near my home. From what those teenagers thought was a game, came an injury that will stay with me for the rest of my life. I was a mile from home, obeying all the rules of the road…it could happen to anyone.

Following the accident the rescue squad rushed me to Inova Fairfax Hospital. When my neurologist told my family I had suffered a moderate diffuse traumatic brain injury, they were devastated. When I finally left the hospital, I did not realize that over the course of a few seconds I lost a life that I had known and loved. I had no idea how long and difficult my journey of recovery would be. I had been a Registered Nurse for 26 years in the same hospital where I was now a patient. I was always the one to care for others, but over the span of these past twelve years, my role has changed from nurse to patient. The reversal of these roles would become one of the most painful parts of my recovery. *I make a much better nurse than I do a patient.*

There were two witnesses that stopped that night. A man traveling behind the teens witnessed the entire race and the accident. When I met him a few months later, he told me he was holding my hands and praying over me as I lay trapped in the car. He said that in those moments, he knew God was not done with me yet, and He had a great plan for me.

Another person stopped to help that night. My husband had been following me home in his own car, and witnessed the entire accident—from the two cars speeding past him, to the impact, to the aftermath that has turned our lives upside down.

During my recovery, he has struggled in his own way. Watching his wife fight an uphill battle against a serious brain injury has been emotionally taxing for him. He is not able to "fix me" like he wishes that he could.

On that day, our oldest daughter was on her way home from the mall with friends at the time of my accident. The police had closed down the parkway, and as they were directing traffic away from them accident, she did that "glance" that we all do. Then she realized that the car in the wreckage was our car. I was told she came running to the car screaming, not knowing what she would find.

I have no outside scars to show you the damage that I have sustained. Doctors call it "the invisible injury." However, I have many torn neurons inside my brain making it hard to *tell* you my journey. Over the next many months, more and more damage was revealed. I was unable to read. I struggled to find words or to form any kind of speech. My memory had vanished. As a nurse I had worked in the NICU, where I was so organized I could make drug calculations in my head, tolerate bright lights, endure constant noise and alarms, and manage life-or-death situations. Now, motion or sound will overwhelm my senses and severely fatigue my brain. I am hyperacusis (increased sensitivity to certain sound/frequency), and can get visually overloaded quickly by simply glancing at a ceiling fan, listening to jazz music, or going out to dinner. I wear special ear filters to decrease the stimuli so that I can function longer before the fatigue sets in, and I then need a nap. They help me to filter what my damaged brain can no longer do.

I like to say I barely survived four long, grueling, painful years of speech, cognitive, and physical therapy. I started by moving my lips to form words, and crawling on the floor to relearn the coordination needed just to improve my walk. My doctors worked diligently with my therapists to put the pieces back together in some form of functioning order. I was not an easy patient. I bounced back and forth between not understanding anything or anyone—to periods of anger, frustration, and depression. The frustration that came from not being able to heal fully, and not being able to reclaim the "old Molly," was a difficult reality to grasp.

In recovery you must get past the realization that you cannot go back to who you once were. Instead, *recovery is knowing how to move forward, to regain the courage that you once had.* I had to grieve for a life I had lost, and be hopeful about the new life I had been given. I had to learn to accept the "new Molly," as did my family and friends.

My family—my husband and two daughters—have all been a huge support to me as we have been learning, struggling, and growing together. I could not have made it this far without their continual love and support. My husband likes to joke that he has done nothing wrong in twelve years because with my speech difficulties, I cannot raise my voice to yell at him. However…he's getting worried as my voice gets stronger.

I was a wife, a mom, and a nurse. I immediately lost my independence, my job, and my ability to do outdoor activities such as skiing, biking, and windsurfing. My children had to care for me. My physical therapist told me that I would never be able to do certain things again. This only fueled the fire within me—I would not let my TBI define my life.

My strong will and determination led me to the National Sports Center for the Disabled (NSCD) in Winter Park, Colorado, where I learned new adaptive skiing methods on the mountain. With my instructors' dedication and encouragement, I heard the words "CAN" instead of "CAN'T." Recently I spent seven weeks out there, and I am using a ski bike. My first goal five years ago was to ride the chair lift. This winter I became completely independent on my ski bike and did double black-diamond runs, moguls, trees, and launched my first jump! I even got some "air time."

In March 2013, while riding the chair lift, I shared my dream with my instructor: to bring combat-wounded veterans to the National Sports Center to benefit from the same life-changing experience I had found in their adaptive sports programs. Shortly thereafter my vision was born. "No Boundaries: Turning Disabilities into Abilities for Our Heroes" was started. It promotes independence, self-esteem, pride, and a sense of accomplishment for all participating combat-wounded veterans.

We fundraise and sponsor a winter and summer program each year that includes an all-expenses-paid trip for ten combat-wounded veterans from across the country. The veterans experience adaptive snow sports in the winter, and whitewater kayaking, rock climbing, and mountain biking in the summer. They benefit from the therapeutic value of living life with other wounded veterans who are facing similar life changes and challenges. "No Boundaries" strives to generate group socialization, camaraderie, and teamwork between the attendees.

On every trip, the staff and veterans are brought to tears as emotional barriers are broken while struggles and stories are shared. At the end of each trip, tears are present again, tears of joy this time, as these veterans look back at the physical and personal growth achievements they've accomplished together.

In my heart, I will always be a nurse. But I also know that I will never practice again. Now, I am helping others in a different way. I feel that the terrible night of my accident was God's plan. And I feel that I have found my purpose: to educate others about this "invisible injury," and to encourage other survivors. In doing so, I, too, now live a life with "no boundaries" anymore.

Molly was a Registered Nurse for 26 years in the NICU before the accident that left her with a TBI. Mike and Molly have two daughters, Ashley, and Lindsay. She loves to go to Colorado to do adaptive sports following her rehab. She is the founder of "No Boundaries: Changing Disabilities into Abilities for Our Heroes," a non-profit organization for combat wounded veterans. Visit our Facebook page: www.facebook.com/noboundariesmilitary

Chapter Sixty-One
TBI: To Become Invincible

**Nick Dennen
Savage, Minnesota**

I was born on Wednesday, April 26, 1978. My life actually began on Sunday, September 27, 1998. Now at age 20, I had experienced a re-birth, a renewal of life. I was born again, not only in the sense of accepting God into my life, but when I discovered my purpose. I had lived 7,459 days not knowing who I was or what I was supposed to do with my life. Mark Twain has said, "The two most important days in your life are the day you are born and the day you find out why."

My "why" arrived in the form of an inspiring message borne from a 35-foot fall, a near drowning, and a two-year rehabilitation. I was at the after-game party, I was drinking with my teammates; I was underage. The party I was at "got busted." I don't remember that night, or the week before, all we know is that a different police officer who was patrolling wanted to investigate what I was doing walking alone at 2:38 a.m. and I was chased by his police dog. So we think trying to escape the dog, I fell off the cliff.

I was unconscious for roughly two months; death was near. My actual time in a coma is questionable, however, even when my eyes opened, I was still completely out of it. I couldn't do anything other than simply lie there. So many people can relate to this pain. Brain injury affects different people in different ways; however, what we share in rehab experience is comparable. Having to relearn certain skills like walking, talking, writing, feeding oneself, brushing one's teeth, or more practical strengths like shopping, organizing data, and making calls to a repair company, do not come easy. In fact, they are practically impossible.

But with physical therapy, occupational therapy, and speech therapy, a person can evolve and become human again. By enduring a TBI, it erases the young person who was once there, the "Old Nick," and begins to construct the new individual who is here now, the "New Nick!" Rebuilding is the key. Yes, you will never be who you were, *but with the right guidance, you can change who you'll become.*

My entire right side was paralyzed for months. I lost over 40 pounds in a matter of a couple months. I was tube fed. I wore diapers. I had to drink thickened liquids. I ate beets, and I hate that disgusting vegetable. I had slurred speech. I had chest tubes. I still have a bald spot on the back of my head showing where my hair fell out. I have a scar on the middle of my throat where the trach was. This is a daily reminder of when life tried (key word here is "tried") to beat me down. My family went through hell not knowing if I would ever get to a point where I could write this story.

What is most unfortunate is how "easy" the media and/or people in general make a recovery from a brain injury seem to be. It does not happen overnight. My rehabilitation took roughly two years, but I can honestly say that it took much longer than that. The "experts" say that recovery from a brain injury is a two-year process. I agree, I was able to start walking, and begin to talk, and perform certain tasks, and go back to school, after a couple years, but I feel that it takes much longer than two years to rebuild and enhance the life that was stolen.

There is a saying that says it takes ten years to become an overnight success. This seems to be more accurate. It also says it take 10,000 hours to become an expert on something—and this averages out to be 20 hours a week for 10 years. With a TBI, this is something we all have "blood memory" of. We have owned every experience, every setback, every loss, every victory, and every lesson we wish we wouldn't have had to learn. We own the pain of our family and friends. So, I think it would be fair to say, that based on these statistics, all of us who experienced our TBI, can be regarded as "experts" on brain injury approximately 417 days after our brains were damaged. Pretty cool, huh?

The critics would disagree. They don't want us to succeed. They don't want us to share our life experience for the greater good. So much of what we have gone through can help other people. So much of our lives can give hope to somebody else. It is more than just surviving a brain injury; it is *thriving because of the brain injury*. It is a way to enhance the healing and develop a stronger version of yourself. The TBI may have ripped our worlds to shreds, but it can be pieced back together through faith, hope, and love.

It is what we experience that can change a life. It is our stories that give strength to an important cause. It is our stories that allow others to share theirs. And it is how we think of our traumatic brain injury that defines us.

TBI is defined as traumatic brain injury. After receiving mine, I have come to realize that TBI has multiple meanings.

1. TBI: To Believe in the Impossible.
2. TBI: To Baffle the Imagination.
3. TBI: To See Beyond the Individual.
4. TBI: To Become Invincible.

David A. Grant, speaker and author of *TBI Hope & Inspiration*, believes TBI means "To Be Inspired." We all need to be inspired. A TBI truly is more than just a traumatic brain injury. It is a life-changing event that tests our strengths, while highlighting our weaknesses. It ultimately comes down to either seeing your glass half-empty, or seeing it as half-full. Initially, I only saw all the things I had lost—the abilities, the future, the life—and wasn't willing to see the things I had won—the new abilities, the new future, the new life. Was it the brain injury preventing me from seeing the bigger picture? Perhaps.

I thought my life was over; I didn't think I was good enough. I thought my brain injury had won. This is all nonsense. It is my hope that reading about my experience will change your perspective, and give you the hope necessary to move forward.

- My balance is off, and I walk with kind of a slight limp at times, but I am walking.
- When I am tired, my speech seems to be a little delayed (probably only to me), but I am talking.

- My right side is still weaker than my left, but I am still able to workout like a house afire at the gym.

So much of what we all experience after enduring a brain injury are experiences that do hold the potential to benefit us. I guess it comes down *to a matter of perspective*, where many of my limitations are self-imposed.

Did I ever think I would ever go through what I had? Heck no! This was something that always happened to somebody else. But once I came to terms with where I was, I was able to see "why" I had been given this knowledge, or opportunity, and what I was supposed to do with it. My former theology professor taught me a theory he developed years ago called, The Dorito Principle. A dorito has three sides. The first side suggests we "Seek to thrive." We can overcome our pains and enhance our life. The second side says, "Seek to love and be loved." We must love others as we love ourselves. And the third side says, "To live for the common good!" Our life's purpose is to make a positive difference in the world. It is never about "us," rather it is about "them," and helping others. I had to redefine TBI.

It is so important to always remember that we are part of something bigger than ourselves. We can make a difference in the world. It's important to remember all the things that we are so extremely fortunate to have. Always recognize that people have feelings—life is too short to hold a grudge—and never be ashamed for the person you are and everything you stand for. Every person matters, and every single life is sacred and deals with its own yesterdays, tomorrows, and todays.

Remember that your attitude will either lift you up, or bring you down, so please make the choice to live your best life now.

Nick Dennen is an inspiring author, speaker, and, first and foremost, a husband and father of two—who would not be here had he not been injured—with a strong purpose of serving the greater good. His mission is to recognize the value of personal relationships while focusing on a positive attitude and heightening the awareness of traumatic brain injury. His motto is simple: anything really is possible if you believe. Anything! www.dennen23.com

Chapter Sixty-Two
Pushing Past Fear

Nikki Abramson
Bloomington, Minnesota

Sharing our deepest personal issues can make us vulnerable, open, and authentic. It is when we are most real with ourselves and with others that we can truly live. While I didn't want to lie to people, I shied away from opening up a part of my story to others. I didn't want to share that I suffered from a traumatic brain injury (TBI). So much stigma already exists around those words. I didn't want people to think of me as less-than, that my brain wasn't working right, that I wasn't "smart" anymore, or that I wasn't capable.

Although my brain isn't able to work like it should, I still am able to pursue important aspects of my life. It has taken time to heal and recover. It has taken time for me to want to, and to be ready, to share my story. I know that when I do open up and share this part of my journey, it can resonate with others, educate, and inspire people in their own life journey—and that is what I am truly all about.

The summer of 2012 was a life-changing time. I was at a weeklong camp where I was a camp counselor of 6th–12th graders at a show-choir camp. I often used a stand-up scooter, the kind that many kids have, but this one was electric. I would zoom around the campus, going from one end of the building to another, making sure that students were at the right place at the right time. Another camp counselor and I were talking as we went back to the dorms while the students were at practice. He walked and I scooted. As we neared the turn to the dorm, I heard a car behind us so I slowed the scooter, and gestured to the driver to pass me so I could go at my own pace. Back on the scooter, I knew I had gripped the handle wrong. I lost my footing, and the scooter went flying from underneath me at 15 mph, crashing me to the cement, face first.

Aaron shouts, "Nikki, Nikki, are you okay?" I brush it off, thinking I am fine. A huge headache comes on, a hematoma the size of a goose egg starts to grow on my forehead, two black-and-blue eyes appear, plus I saw blood from my skinned-up knees and elbows that also took a beating. Aaron walked the scooter back to the dorm only a few feet away; then he found me something to sit on, so he could run to get ice and call 911, my parents, and our camp directors.

Aaron rushed me in his van to the nearest ER. I remember he kept talking to me and making sure I was okay. I kept saying, "Aaron, I am fine. Let's go back. The kids need us." I go in and out of consciousness. Aaron stays with me as we wait our turn to see a doctor. At this point the headache is beyond anything I can even describe. I am in so much pain I can barely see straight. My eyes are swollen. Blood continues to pour out of parts of my body, and the goose egg bump continues to grow and grow.

The camp director stops by while I am having MRI. My parents and I talked on the phone to make sure I am okay. "Yes, Dad, I think I am okay. I will see how I feel in the morning and maybe see my primary doctor." They x-rayed my face and brain to make sure that my brain is okay. It turns out things were okay, and that originally I had a headache, was nauseous, and looked horrible for that week. I was on pain medication. The doctor told me, "You might have some side effects because you took a hard landing to your head and brain, but you should be okay. Take this medication." I ask if I can continue to stay at camp or if I need to stay at home. "You can go to camp if your able to be okay, but rest and take it easy." This was just day one of camp. I was devastated, yet fought it out.

Weeks later, I still had these headaches. I was forgetting things; in fact, I couldn't remember anything, like how to do simple tasks. I felt horrible. I ended up seeing another doctor who then diagnosed a TBI. TBI, I thought to myself...I don't need another condition. I was then sent to speech therapy and occupational therapy to help my attention, focus, and concentration skills.

Therapy was a long-and-hard battle. At the time, I was also in graduate school trying to pursue my master's degree. I couldn't read for long periods of time without getting headaches. The words on the page would be jumbled together and become foggy. I forgot things, and had to have checklists everywhere. I ended up taking time off school because it was too hard on my brain. Watching TV, a simple task that normally relaxed my brain, was stressful on my brain. Being on the computer would be so taxing on my brain, and for several months, I would barely be able to respond to a few emails here and there.

When the doctor recommended that I attend speech therapy, I was offended. I can speak fine and have no difficulty with coming up with words. I didn't want to tell people I was going to speech therapy because then, I'd get questions like, "You speak fine, why are you in speech?" The speech therapist helped me to break down daunting items. I remember trying to do my laundry, and the tasks, like cooking a simple meal, were too hard to break down in my head. She gave me tools for how to organize my schedule and calendar with to-do lists and color-coding, as well as learning to advocate for myself. I also got a Lumosity subscription where I could play games online every day to help my brain build up to where it used to be. I continued this subscription, and now four years later, Lumosity still helps me. I am grateful for these tools that I have been given that I still use so I can continue to help the symptoms of this difficult condition.

Recovery is a process. In many ways, I have recovered from TBI; however, in other ways I feel as though I am still recovering. It has been life changing, and I think I will always recover in other ways. The biggest obstacle in suffering from with TBI is the fact that people say, "You look fine. You look better, you must be feeling better." I wanted others to know about this invisible condition of my brain. *I wanted people to live with my brain just for a day, to see how difficult it was for me. It was like my world was upside down.*

Another obstacle I faced was loss. Losing my ability to do things made me discouraged. It made me feel inadequate, not good enough, and more importantly, I didn't feel like myself. A little piece of me was missing—my brain. Some days I couldn't think; it hurt my brain to think. To plan out my day was overwhelming and exhausting, a task I normally enjoy and love.

I didn't want to tell others that I suffered from a TBI because I was fearful about what people would think of me. I worked hard in my life to get to where I am. I didn't want people to see me as weak. I didn't want people to look at me as though I couldn't do anything. To those of us that suffer, many others in this world have also gone through this. It is not fun. You are not alone. Hang in there. Take it one day at a time.

Some days I didn't think I would ever regain the ability to be on the computer, read, or watch TV. I have worked hard to be able to do what I can do. I have taken the time to quiet down my mind, and accept where I am. It is okay. It is okay to accept where you are.

There is always HOPE. Life is hard, and you never know what might be thrown at you. Yet there is always hope. Don't ever give up on this. Keep seeking out answers. I remember seeing a few different doctors and therapists and tried numerous options to see what might work. One thing would work for someone else, but not for me. You just never know. Be patient and kind to yourself. I was fearful of what others would think of me. I have learned to accept myself and who I am, *TBI and all.*

Self-care and self-love are the greatest gifts you can give yourself. You are loved. There is hope. Hold on!

Nikki Abramson is the author of the books "I Choose Hope" in 2014 and "Hope for Today" in 2016, as well as co-author for a one hour one-woman play, "No Limits." She is a teacher, actor, speaker, and mentor who strives to bring hope and positivity to the world specifically in the areas of disabilities and adoption. Check out NikkiAbramson.com for more information on her story and work.

Chapter Sixty-Three
Dakota Strong

Nita Massey
Carrabelle, Florida

August 4, 2015 started off like any other normal day in our lives. I was a sergeant at Franklin Correctional Institution, a maximum-security State men's prison in the Florida panhandle. I worked the nightshift. Our youngest son, Dakota, was an officer and worked the dayshift. I remember Dakota calling to tell me he was going on a transport, which means transporting an inmate. In this case the inmate had completed his sentence, and Dakota was taking him to a bus station in Tallahassee Florida to go home to his family. Like always, I told him to be careful and that I loved him. Little did I know it would be the last time I heard his voice.

At approximately 3:15 p.m., my son's Ford Taurus and a semi met head on at a curve ten miles from home. I remember the institution calling my husband, telling us that Dakota had been in a wreck. We immediately jumped up and ran out the door as soon, falling in behind the ambulance. When we got to the scene and saw the semi and Dakota trapped inside his car, we realized just how bad it was.

Dakota was unconscious inside the car, and I could see a very spiritual coworker in the backseat, and I knew she was praying over my baby. Our colonel and another officer were keeping me away from the car because they already knew how critical Dakota was. The first three people on scene were a doctor, a nurse, and an EMT, all from out of state, who had been down on the coast visiting. To us, God knew exactly what he was doing that day, and He put people in place so that we would not lose our son.

Dakota suffered a traumatic brain injury, and a fracture in the neck at the brain stem, which thankfully was centimeters away from a more devastating injury, and healed on its own with twelve weeks of neck stabilization. He also had two fractures in his back, a broken femur, and a broken hip. Due to the airbag's force, Dakota's whole face was a maze of fractures, and his jaw was broken. We were given little hope that he would survive surgery, or even survive the 72-hour mark. We were also told that if he did live, he would remain in a vegetative state for the rest of his life.

Dakota has continued to fight and prove the doctors wrong. In February 2016 Dakota was reclassified to "a minimally conscious state." That April we almost lost Dakota again when an infection in his abdomen traveled up the tubing to his shunt into his brain. Dakota fought this battle, and after 53 days, we brought him home once again.

I want Dakota's story to bring faith and peace that with God all things are possible. Although at this time Dakota does not talk or walk, we and his wonderful therapist are very hopeful that in time he will conquer and win in these areas as well. In the past two weeks, it is like Dakota is at a whole new level, and is showing emotions. We see his beautiful smile almost every day now, and we are forever thankful for all of the prayers we have received as a family.

My word of advice to other parents going through similar situations is to never give up as God is our ultimate healer.

No bio provided.

Chapter Sixty-Four
The Gift of a Near-Fatal Fall

Pamela Leigh Richards
Sedona, Arizona

It has been almost seven years since my fall on January 24, 2010. A day I will always hold onto as one of the greatest gifts that life could have given me. Indeed life is a personal journey for all of us, and so here I share a moment in time. The gods were surely on my side this day.

I fell twelve feet from the loft in the garage, slipping from the top rung of the ladder straight onto concrete. I landed completely on my left side, fracturing my skull, and suffering a subcutaneous hematoma, head trauma with left epidural hematoma, cerebral contusions, hairline fracture of spine, fractured left wrist, nine rib fractures, and had bruising all over my left side. The last thing I remember is sitting on the ledge. Then time passed me by, without a clue.

Somehow I got up in a lucid state and walked across the courtyard of the main property where I rented a tiny glass guesthouse. No one was in the main house at the time so I was completely alone. How I opened a sliding glass door with nine broken ribs, found my way to the bed where I laid down basically to die, is in and of itself surreal. Maybe heaven bent a wee bit and held my hand so I would not lose everything. The outside world was happening; however, I was somewhere inside beyond reach.

What happened next was truly a miracle. My landlords were in town across the valley at one of their other properties when the wife felt a strong urge, an intuitive nudge telling her to "go back to the property!" She told her husband she had to go, which she did, thank goodness.

Walking to the guesthouse she knocked on the sliding glass door, heard my moaning and immediately entered to find me lying on the bed. In retrospect, it's interesting that all doors were left unlocked. If she had not listened to that "message" and come back on that sunny Sunday afternoon, I would not be writing this.

My next awareness was opening my eyes slightly, and in a blurred vision I recognized blood was all over my white comforter before going unconscious again. The wife tried to get me in the car, but I did not want to go. Somehow I pulled myself to sit up on the bed, feet on the floor, but as I stood, I immediately threw up before falling back on the bed. So now there was blood and vomit all over the place. The woman did not know what to do, so she called her husband on the cell phone. The next thing I remember briefly is a voice shouting, "She's going to die! Call 911!" before losing consciousness again. I found out later that I was hearing her husband over the phone's speaker. He had been an ER doctor, and soon made his way over. The Sedona Fire Department responded to the emergency call, and the ball started rolling.

Five paramedics were managing a very serious situation, but I was completely in a long-gone state. One of the paramedics began sleuthing, following a trail of blood from the glass house to the garage, discovering blood on the floor under the loft next to the ladder. He realized I must have fallen. I found out later when I asked what happened, they said I kept moaning and pulling my left wrist, so they cut off my long sleeves, exposing the break. Shortly thereafter I was carried on a stretcher to the ambulance, which took me to the Sedona Medical Center where the extent of my injuries were discovered. I was immediately flown by helicopter north to Flagstaff Medical Center for emergency brain surgery.

I had two neurosurgeons working on me first. They made an incision from the top of my head straight down to just below my left ear. I was told a circle of my skull was cut out and removed around the fracture line so they could drain the blood from my brain. They then placed this circular piece of skull back in and secured it with four tiny titanium plates and screws. I later said I am now a walking GPS!

Once I was stable, the orthopedic surgeon performed his skills on my fractured wrist as a metal plate was inserted to hold the bone together for healing. I also had staples in my head from the top to bottom securing it in place. My neurologist told me that my injury was in one of the most dangerous places it could have been in. When he showed the images, it was very revealing. The hematoma (blood buildup) was squashing the left part of my brain inward. If it had grown and pressed just slightly further, we are talking a fraction of an inch, it would have hit the brain stem, which means no transmission and lights out for Pamela, instantly. The gods were on my side for sure that day. I am very grateful for the love and care I received from everyone who helped.

When I awoke in hospital there was no one familiar, only hospital staff who became my family. I was simply lying down in ICU in a room with people who were caring for me in the beginning stages of recovery.

On some level I was completely out of my body. However, it was peaceful wherever I was, somewhere I couldn't explain. Maybe the morphine was coming to my rescue when necessary? You won't know until you get there, and the language of man will never be able to describe the indescribable. My body was in pain, and only when I awoke in the hospital room, did the pain of nine broken ribs reveal themselves *loud and clear.*

Just before I was released they asked if I wanted to try and take a shower, and I said yes. Wow! What an experience. The nurse walked me to the shower and left. It was the strangest feeling, but I was able to undress and stand in the shower for a brief moment of cleaning. Then it hit. I became very dizzy, nauseous, lost coordination, and began crying for help as I drifted in a slow fall onto the wooden bench. The nurse had to help me dress and get me back to my room to lie down. I did not want to leave the hospital.

After two weeks I was released. The very kind nurse brought me to the front doors of the hospital in a wheelchair. Oh to see the Sun, feel winter's gentle breeze, and to smell the great northern air was a pure delight! Time to go home for further rest and recovery, and I was as ready as I would ever be.

The only family I have left is my elderly father. He came to visit one time but he was in early stages of Alzheimers. So, no one was there to pick me up except a taxi. The drive was surreal as I viewed the forests alongside the road, for it simply made every cell in my body sing with a new recognition of it. I became one with everything. It was so beautiful. I could have sat there forever watching in bliss. I truly was one of the lucky ones.

My beloved father had arranged for a caregiver, who was waiting for me at the house. This amazing lady, Patty, will forever hold a very special place in my heart. She would come and go as necessary, making sure I had food and nourishment, and took me to doctor appointments. I remember the day Patty and I decided it was time for me to take a shower. She washed me down, wrapped me up, and sat me in a chair where she spent at least an hour combing all the tangles out of my hair. I can't tell you how good that felt.

I stopped all morphine and sleeping pills in about a month. Yes, I was still in pain, as I lay in bed for months, watching the world go by through my sliding glass door into my magic garden. In order to get up, I had to roll over onto my right side, use my right arm to lift up, then was able to stand up from the bed.

In the beginning stages of recovery, I laughingly shared views that sprang forth in a sort of philosophical manner. It is just the way I saw the world as I woke up, seeing with new eyes, in the sense that if one part of my brain closed (left logical), other parts opened and lit up (right creativity). Therefore, I had a new view of everything. Nature was talking to me, and I became very connected to it. The wind, the leaves on the trees, the birds singing, the Earth beneath my feet, the flowers growing so gently at a pace in peace, it was all speaking to me without thinking. I was operating from my heart brain, not my head brain.

With the gift of this fall, my life changed directions in a manner of grace.

From a biological or artistic point of view, I see some reasoning as to why I saw differently. Is it possible that having the left side of my brain squashed, might have caused the neurons in that part of the brain to stop firing from a transmitter to a receiver? They are called neural nets that form through repeating environments, creating our habits, behaviors, addictions, etc. When the environment changes, those neural nets, habits, addictions, behaviors, literally unplug because they don't have the familiar reaction they once had, therefore every cell is now awaiting new instruction as it falls away.

Symbolically, a few books of memory in the library of my brain were not receiving a connection; therefore, certain memories once stored were now gone. Reminds me of the burning of the Library of Alexandria, Egypt. This is why I would say after the fall, "The chatter doesn't matter." It was such a freeing feeling to let go of most thought, which is what happened to me. I began to scan the world and "know it," vs. literalize it. I woke up having no thought, at least in areas that were irrelevant, in my view, at this point. It was as if my mind became free, and fear was removed.

For me the outside world was not fitting my inside one, with confusion on both sides, and a wish to go deeper into the *hows* and *whys* to help us all heal. What I have learned as well, is that in order for us to get over our fears, or sufferings of any kind, we must put a stop sign on every moment, on every corner where a thought enters, trying to get you to go down a habitual road that needs deleting so you can think clearly without interference. Only you will know when to hold that sign up and walk another way, knowing you are so not alone, and that you can do it unafraid.

This challenge was, and still is, an ongoing discovery of the awe of life and our connections with it. We dip in, we dip out, we come, we go—all an inevitable equation. I simply want to make the journey peaceful with love and care, and may we all go out on our own terms, not someone or something else's.

This fall was an experience that propelled me further into understandings I have held deep "within," probably since beyond my birth, which are now blossoming. It is a Gift of Life I shall not waste. It is like a closed window now opening. I am ever so grateful.

> "Sometimes you have to die, in order to wake up."
> – Pamela Leigh Richards

Some of my friends with TBIs would say they never really want to mention they have a TBI when in public situations. I come from another position. When I was talking with customer service representatives on the phone while trying to pay a bill, or get information, or ordering at a restaurant, depending on the circumstances, I would say: "I have a TBI, so could you please speak slowly." The compassion immediately comes through and they apologize, especially after I share what a TBI is, and the brief of my story. Everyone I have freely opened up to, become amazed. It is just one more person being aware. Every time we do this, we teach about the *silent epidemic*, opening the door of communication with others, letting them know they are not alone, and to be more compassionate. This for me is the awakening—the awakening of not being afraid to share your stories.

> "Say what you were ever afraid to say.
> Listen, when you did not think you ever would.
> Slow down your breathing before ever speaking.
> Love the very thing you felt your heart never could.
> Look where thine eyes feared to seek.
> Embrace All with forgiveness and understandings.
> And in the end, merging into New Beginnings.
> This shall be a mighty fine relief."
> – Pamela Leigh Richards

Pamela is an artist of living, author, photographer, filmmaker, philosopher, poet, creative director, dancer, and lover of all things nurturing nature's coherent elegance. She grew up in Europe and has travelled the world, with an English/Norwegian lineage. Since her TBI she woke up seeing with new eyes, which ignited a soulful purpose, shifting her life towards a fascination of physics and how life works, and what are we doing here? She is still assimilating.

Chapter Sixty-Five
In a Blink of An Eye: Life After Brain Injury

Paul Bosworth
Lafayette, Louisiana

I grew up in an area known for its food, hospitality, and music, where the natives could be ready for a party within a moment's notice—New Orleans, Louisiana. At a very early age, I learned to cook because you have to serve food at parties, right? My knack for learning and being prepared would serve me well in life. I had been selling ladies shoes for fourteen years, which taught me to do the dance for sales, but doing so slowly grew old. I acquired my college degree at Louisiana State University (LSU) later in life; then went into sales for a leading company's personal computing division, which was later acquired by another cutting-edge company.

In my forties, I was finally living my dream. Everything had clicked into place as I had found a role where I could explore my untapped talents. I was happy growing my business in the Washington, DC territory, and I loved many things about the area: happy hours, thriving energy, the Washington Nationals, and its history and culture. There was always something to do.

On Tuesday, September 11, 2007, the company's inside sales team in Raleigh, North Carolina set up a call with a client to discuss an opportunity that was worth millions—and I was learning the background, shape, and size of the client's business. While working alone in my home office, I was eating some chicken fried rice. I choked hard on a bite of food, and the world went black as the thought shot across my mind, "This is not good!"

When I fell, my dream life made an immediate exit.

Apparently, I got up from my desk, phone set to ring, instant messenger open, and email pinging away on my ThinkPad as I staggered sideways, sort of falling into my tiny kitchen a few feet away. Lunch had become lodged tightly in my throat, and oxygen to my brain was cut off. I passed out, smacking my head on the floor, and perhaps also against the dishwasher as well as other hard surfaces. Apparently, all my choking and thrashing about on the tiny kitchen floor had knocked my lunch just free enough to allow air to reenter my lungs, albeit laboriously. I could not see clearly, as if I was looking through slivered glass. I was shaking uncontrollably, trying to get back up. I needed to get rid of this food stuck in my throat.

Wheezing, I blinked continuously to see my way to my bathroom in order to clear the jammed food loose. I popped the food out by gagging, ripping my throat in four places—and there was a lot of blood. I could breathe, but I was very scared, and was crying, shaking, and I could not see straight. And, I was missing the sales call.

I reached my desk and had to tilt my head down to focus my eyes. I "instant messaged" the team manager, telling him what happened. He kept typing, "Go to the hospital." I obstinately ignored his plea since I simply *had to be on this call*. His message repeated several times, hence my memory of it. I called my girlfriend. Why should I call 911? I just conked my head and ripped up my throat. So what? I should be fine.

I had no clue that my life just turned down a very dark, lonely path. I learned later that few people really know how to deal with a concussion.

My girlfriend picked my bruised, blinded, and disoriented self from the parking lot in front of my apartment to bring me to the Virginia Hospital Center just minutes away. I was treated and released on September 11, 2007, complete with a copious amounts of pain killers. I was in pain as well as quite combative, belligerent, and incoherent as I had lost my best asset—my ability to communicate.

Both the nurse and the attending ER doctor strongly lectured my increasingly frightened girlfriend about what to do with me. The doctor possessed a snarky, condescending tone, stating: "This may all just go away, but we are really not sure," which made my demeanor much worse. What do you mean by "not sure"? Valium was added to my stack of medications to take me down a notch. On that day in September of 2007, the hospital *had no protocol* to admit me. My girlfriend was completely responsible for me now, and she cared wonderfully for me.

Later a therapist figured my mTBI (mild traumatic brain injury) registered about an 8 or 9 on the Glasgow Coma Scale. Without going into a technical definition, a mild traumatic brain injury sounds much like a conk on the head that will just go away, however mine was more serious, yet I am classified as "mild." In my view, medical science has some redefining to do.

Doctors went straight to work stopping the bleeding in my throat. But, they had few methods to treat the concussion. Concussions just fade away, right? *I was ashamed* to admit that I have so many symptoms from just conking my head. My symptoms would alight like butterflies; then seemingly fly away. I had many expensive tests to no avail. I went to many doctors, always ending up at the front of the line. I recall boasting loudly with my now missing filter, "Boy, this is great! Who doesn't wait in the doctor's office? This guy!"

Organs began misfiring. My heart randomly malfunctioned, so I went to the best cardiology group. No kidding, I would urinate about 50–60 times a day, so I saw the best urologist. My sleep was affected, so add another doctor to the list. My eye, the one I saw "slivered" scenes through, got me to the best neuro eye doctor who talked really fast, plus another in Georgetown, DC who kept staring into her scope, perplexed, saying, "Your eye is normal, but when light catches, it shows microscopic cracks…I've never seen this before." Great, I thought, "My life is over." When my girlfriend took me to my numerous doctors' visits, these were our dates. Sleep was tricky because often I would relive the accident.

Those closest to me categorically *would not accept* that "I had a brain injury." This went on for months.

After dozens of appointments, and the promise that using catheters to drain me was the plan, I threw out most of my medications. I shared this news with my cutting-edge, understanding neurologist who diagnosed me in minutes with "post-concussion syndrome." Talk about luck! We had met months before my injury at a happy hour and discussed a popular jazz festival. He committed to help me deal and cope, as best as he could. My connections to a local TBI

Program at INOVA (Infirmary of Northern Virginia) in Mount Vernon began with him. Upon graduating, I obtained contact information from my speech therapist. I collected contacts of everyone who understood mTBI (mild traumatic brain injury). Was there a way out? My speech therapist connected me to Brain Injury Services (BIS). BIS assured me that there was life ahead of me, as they are the voice in the storm.

Surely, there was someone who had a clue on helping to heal my brain. I lived to think outside the box. In 2012, I was back to Googling, and found someone. The doctor lived and helped brains in New Orleans, my hometown. I was invited to his reception/talk in New Orleans. So, I jumped on a plane to visit my friends. Due to the overwhelming interest, the reception lasted only 10 minutes before he segued directly into his talk. He referenced applying oxygen to a wound under pressure to awaken brain cells after trauma. He gave example after example of those who have benefitted so far. I needed to take important notes as his work would be game changing.

I remember what he said to me with a smile, "I think I can help you feel better." My heart swelled as my answer resembled, "Let's do this!"

I brought my notes back home and researched this Hyperbaric Oxygen Therapy (HBOT) for months. Then, luckily, I cold-called a local HBOT doctor who was up to date on this simple concept. I made a cash deal using my inheritance, and within a year had completed my first forty treatments, known as dives. The brain is slow to heal, so eventually, for the first time in five years, I walked away with evidence of substantial concussion from a PET/CT brain scan as well as an improved quality of life. I am not 100 percent, *but I am better*.

Remember the frequent urinating? After I completed the HBOT dives, I began neurofeedback treatments. Within a week, it reduced the number of bathroom trips to a normal range.

In August 2010, I saved up enough energy to attend a support group in my new hometown of Lafayette, Louisiana. I created a "bucket system" that I apply daily. If my sleep bucket is low, then my symptoms will show up. So, fill my sleep bucket and I am going to act normal for a few hours. Fill my food bucket if I am going somewhere and will need stamina. A few hours before I go to a party I need to get some quiet time.

So, I went to the local support group meeting, yet no one was around for the meeting. Sitting near me was a very popular woman greeting the healthcare workers passing in the lobby. After 15 minutes, I asked if she knew anything about the TBI meeting. She said she was running it, but no one had shown up yet. My face lit up. "Hi! I'm Paul. I'm here for the meeting. I am a survivor." She looked at me with a surprised look and said, "Oh, I would have never known...." My face showed that my hope for support was dashed, as I felt deep sadness and hopelessness. No TBI survivor *ever* wants to hear these words.

Within an hour, I vowed to find a way to educate those who matter so that this would never happen again—even if it takes forever.

Today, I moderate a brain injury support group that just celebrated six years. If you bring people together to talk about a common topic, somebody will be helped. We call our group AMAZE, and we meet primarily to make sure no one with a TBI is alone. I spend time coaching people on a one-to-one basis as much as I am able. I also give talks and pitch in to help with a local BBQ to support Brain Injury Awareness. I gain brain back every time I use my brain, as long as I nurture it afterwards with whole foods, rest, and water. The more I use my brain for good intentions, the happier I am.

Volunteering is key therapy in bringing my brain back. I have found that sitting in the past beckons depression and bad decisions, just as drinking alcohol and drugs make matters worse. Like many of us, I carried a substantial amount of shame post-injury, and comfort food is readily available to salve the pain, thus I gained weight. Since then, I have learned to release pain, and grab hold of something worthwhile: LIFE.

For me, sharing my insights with any size group is impactful. It gets me up and out to share my story for this "silent epidemic." More importantly, I can deliver talking points such as: 1) brain injury is a leading cause of death and disability in the US; or, 2) by midnight tonight over 6,000 people will sustain a brain injury; or, 3) every 13 seconds someone in America sustains a brain injury. These statistics are increasing as awareness grows.

By visiting Capitol Hill, DC, in March, I learned about HBOT, neurofeedback, biomarkers, a small app to detect concussion, and why whole foods and music are my favorite "drugs." Our military has taken the lead in generating protocol for brain injury. History shows that the NFL has a high rate of concussions and suicides, especially in retirees.

You are not alone!

Once I stopped waiting for a drug to bring back my brain, options came into view as I found the low-hanging fruit was there all along: volunteering, essential oils, veggie juicing, HBOT, and other therapies that lead to strategies for brain improvement. Every brain is different. Social media has groups that help. Remember, sugar short-circuits my brain and invites depression, protein is powerful, and naps are necessary. Meditation helps daily. Walking gets the blood flowing, which brings oxygen to the brain.

I am here to help the next person thrive. My hope is that you keep going every day, and take ownership of your brain, enabling it to work better. My career making millions in sales is history; however, today sharing my story affects millions of brain cells for the next Survivor. In my moment of great loss, I found myself. Keep an eye out for my book, to be launched in 2017, as I go into detail about the topics I mentioned here. *Awareness Is Growing*!

Paul G Bosworth is an expert survivor, writer, advocate, BBQ guy, brain injury support group moderator, and public speaker. He is influencing others to gain back brain cells through non-traditional means, including hyperbaric oxygen therapy. He sits on the State of Louisiana Traumatic Head Injury/Spinal Cord Injury Trust Fund Program Board and Brain Injury Association of America's Brain Injury Advisory Council. He promotes Smoky Breaux's BBQ for Brain Injury fundraiser held yearly in Cajun Country. A Brain Injury focused non-profit is in the works as well. Paul goes the distance to advocate for the overwhelmed millions of Americans dealing with this silent epidemic. His message of hope starts in his backyard and goes throughout the world.

Chapter Sixty-Six
Waiting for the Silver Lining

Rebecca Hannam
Fergus, Ontario, Canada

One snowy Sunday in February 2008 changed my life forever—but it took eight years for the realization to come full circle.

I was participating in a horseback-riding lesson, keen to train for what would have been my first show season. We had an ice storm the previous day, and sheets of white were atop every building in sight. As the morning sun came out and the temperature warmed, the ice began to melt, and as it slid off the arena roof, the noise spooked my horse. I remember hearing my coach instructing me to regain control, but Simon, my lesson horse, was too fast and too wild. Flying around the arena is the last thing I remember from that day and the three that followed.

I was thrown off Simon, and unfortunate timing led me straight into the wooden arena door frame. I hit the left side of my head, cracked my helmet open and injured my shoulder. I was knocked unconscious from the hit, and an ambulance was called to the farm. At the hospital I had many tests, and my family and I were told that my helmet saved my life. I was discharged with a diagnosis of a concussion, and was instructed to schedule physiotherapy for my shoulder. No other guidance was provided, and I was sent home to rest.

The following days were spent resting while loved ones stopped in for visits—none of which I remembered. It was the winter of my grade 12 (senior) year, and while I did spend a few school days at home, I returned to life as I knew it shortly after. I worked with a well-respected physiotherapist, and within a few months my shoulder's mobility improved significantly.

The following September, I attended university and lived on campus, and quickly filled my time with extracurricular and volunteer involvements. Although I was learning about an industry I am passionate about, my mind often had doubts about my program decision. I would lie in my dorm room, crying without any trigger. Classes became difficult, and despite reading, re-reading and re-reading again, studying didn't seem to stick. My grades dropped dramatically from those in high school, but I chalked it up to the new experience—and I didn't tell anyone about these challenges. University was supposed to be hard, right?

Things improved with time, and by my final year I was leading a student marketing team, working as a freelance writer on campus, sitting on two boards of directors, and receiving offers for full-time positions. I also held a healthy attendance record at campus pubs, and loved nothing more than singing and dancing at our local country bar.

Post-convocation/graduation I started a career in financing and continued to stay busy with industry and community commitments. While my concussion hadn't been talked about in years, I often experienced headaches and neck pain. Every once in a while I would see a physiotherapist to get checked out, and they always said that it was neck, shoulder and jaw tension, and often implied that this was a result of the stressful, busy life I led.

In May 2015 I was suddenly hit with nausea, dizziness, constant headaches, and a ringing sound in my ears that I had never heard before. My family doctor, the same one who barely discussed my concussion with me seven years prior, was confident that I was experiencing stress burnout and *recommended anti-depressant medication*. I tried the medication, but as the symptoms stayed constant for the next month, my gut told me it must be something more. At my next appointment she informed me that "I was complaining," and should go to see a therapist to help me relax. That advice didn't sit well with me, and after switching doctors, my new assessment resulted in a leave of absence from work, and led to what seemed like every scan and test in the book.

I was, of course, very hesitant to take a leave of absence, but my doctor must have seen people like me before, as he did not give me a choice—but rather sent his instructions to my employer. With each and every test I hoped that "something" would be found, but instead I became more and more disappointed. Findings of "normal" are supposed to make people happy, but to me it was dreadful news. The symptoms were wasting my time; it was time to be able to do more than work on my laptop from bed with ice packs on my head.

Five months went by before I was allowed to gradually restart office hours, and even then, I did not feel like myself. My new family doctor continued to refer me to specialists in hopes of finding a way to solve the symptom mystery. I asked to be referred to an ear specialist to see if anything could be done for my tinnitus. In the doctor's waiting room I filled out the forms telling the story of my ear ringing. When she entered the appointment room she looked at me from different angles before saying, "You have had a concussion and/or whiplash on the left side. When was it?" My jaw dropped.

This doctor was the first person to connect my symptoms to my past concussion, and this lead to seeing a physiotherapist and dentist who specialize in head injuries. The concussion team was shocked that I had finished high school and university without delay and that I held the positions I did. My symptoms started to improve under their care, but I was still very focused on getting my life back.

One evening in February 2016, just two business days before I was allowed to return to work full-time again, one of the worst case scenarios played out. I slipped on my front walkway and hit the back of my head perfectly square on the corner of my cement step. I tried to ignore it, but eventually ended up in the emergency room. I was diagnosed with another concussion, and to my surprise, this ER doctor had a full page of protocol notes to follow—*and a handout of instructions for me to take home.*

This only eight years later, all I could think of was how differently my earlier fall from the horse would have been treated if it happened now.

Even though all of the symptoms I was previously experiencing got worse, and some new ones were added to the list by my fall on the ice, I know it is teaching me the life lessons I was probably supposed to learn the first time. The advancement in concussion research is amazing, and I continue to see parallels between the now-known concussion symptoms and my past experiences.

As I write this (an activity that is requiring more effort, breaks and editing than ever before), I am on a long-term injury leave from work. I am seeing a concussion doctor, physiotherapist, massage therapist, and vision therapist weekly. I currently suffer from head pain and pressure, neck tension, tinnitus, dizziness, fatigue, light and noise sensitivity and short-term memory loss. While I've seen improvement, it is a very slow process. It is also a lonely process, and *I will openly admit there are days when it is hard to find joy.*

It is still unknown if I will be able to return to the type of job I was doing, resume my freelance business, or even to what level some of my symptoms will improve, but I do know this experience has changed my life. The second fall acted like a forced timeout, as instantly I had to give up my job and almost all of my involvements. But it has also has taught me about the value of self-care and the importance of gratitude in a way I would have never slowed down long enough to learn.

Here's my new perspective: On two different occasions, I have hit my head so hard that I could have died. I'm still here, and there must be a reason for that. While I don't yet know what I am meant to do with my life from this point on, or even when I am going to be able to leave the house without sunglasses, ear plugs, and being in constant pain, I know that it will be carried out at a calmer, more sustainable pace with healthier habits and greater faith.

Rebecca Hannam is an agriculture communications professional based in Fergus, Ontario, Canada. Find her on Twitter @rebeccahannam.

Chapter Sixty-Seven
I Am a Fighter

Renie Bania
West Rutland, Vermont

On April 25th, 2015, my girlfriend (who I'll call Mary), and I were heading about two hours away to her sister's house to have dinner out on the town, with her sister and her wife. It was kind of cool, but a nice afternoon for a spring day. On our drive there, we laughed and listened to music. When we got there we were greeted with smiles. Mary remembered that she had a set of china dishes in her sister's garage, so we started discussing whether she was going to put them in the Jeep Cherokee—and if she should back up the Jeep, or leave it where it was because the dishes were heavy.

I have bad hearing and did not realize Mary was backing up the jeep so I continued to walk towards the back of the garage. That's when her foot slipped off the brake, hitting the gas and accelerating. We are not sure if she hit me, or it was the two upright freezers on the back wall of the garage. The Jeep's speed caused the freezers to fall on top of me, and everything inside came out on top of me. My body was underneath the freezer, but my head was sticking out.

Mary's sister was moving her car out of the garage and came running to lift the freezer off me as much as she could. Mary crawled under the freezer to make sure I was alive. She asked me what hurt, and I keep saying, "My head, my head," as I was bleeding across my entire forehead. She said that her back hurt, knowing I would hold her and not touch my head anymore.

I don't remember anything that was said or done after that. The back of my head was fractured in the shape of a V, my leg was torn open and my knee was broken in half, and my elbow was bleeding, but it was a superficial wound.

While I was in the hospital for two weeks, my family got me to sign a paper for a lawyer, wanting me to sue Mary. Of course, I did not know what I was signing. My family also told friends and other family that Mary tried to kill me on purpose. Some of her family insisted she was on drugs, including her sister. She has over twenty years of recovery, and helps other women on a daily basis. When I became somewhat aware of what was going on, I called the lawyer from the hospital, and stopped it.

The day after I was released from the hospital, my mother had my aunt come in her camper to make sure she got me out of the state away from Mary. Mom drove my car and my aunt drove me in the camper down to Florida, many miles from where I lived in Vermont.

I was 45 at the time of the accident. I had no health insurance down there, no doctors, and no medical care. I was depressed, lonely and had no one to trust or talk to. I still talked to Mary. Three months later, I decided I had had enough, and drove back to Vermont by myself. Yes, it was dangerous, but "someone" was watching out for me. I had been having seizures, but didn't have any on the way home, making it home just fine.

Mary got me the best medical care I could possibly get— three neurologists, and a primary doctor, and I started speech, occupational, and physical therapy, which I finished this year. I was behind because I did not get the help I needed at the beginning. I do not talk to some of my family today. I will keep on going, trying to figure out who the new me is, and what my new place in life will be. I will not let the TBI define who I am. Yes, I am different now, but I will find my place in life because I don't give up. I can be who I want to be with hard work and dedication. My new puppy, Blaze, will be trained to be a service dog, and she's also my best friend. I AM A FIGHTER.

Renie lives in West Rutland, Vermont. She is an avid UCONN Huskies fan. Renie loves spending time with her friend and her new puppy, Blaze.

Chapter Sixty-Eight
Our Recovery Never Stops

Ric Johnson
Minneapolis, Minnesota

In case you're wondering, falls are the main cause of brain injuries, and I'm living proof.

On Saturday, October 18, 2003, I was fifty-three-years-old and in perfect health. I was cleaning the gutters on my house, a household task I did for twenty-plus years. I finished and stepped on a ladder to get down from the roof. And down I went. Seems that I missed the first step, and landed on a concrete slab on the driveway. My 13-year-old daughter saw me fall, and that I didn't standup. She ran over, and discovered I was unconscious. Fortunately she called 911 and waited for an ambulance. I was rushed to the Hennepin County Medical Center (HCMC) in Minneapolis. Since only our daughter and I were at home at that time, she went with me in the ambulance, and called home to tell my wife that I fell and was "at the hospital," but forgot to say which hospital. My wife, Beth, came home, listened to the message, spent a few minutes trying to find which hospital, and drove over as soon as she knew.

When Beth arrived, she found me in the Brain Injury Intensive Care Unit, restrained, surrounded by nurses and doctors, with machines and tubes keeping me alive. Beth called our son, telling him what happened. He arrived a few hours later, and they all spent the rest of the night, waiting for details. There were no details. Staff only said I was in critical condition. They spent the following day, Sunday, in the waiting room calling family members about my injury. Family members started arriving, asking for news, but again, it was only that I was still in critical condition.

On the following Thursday my wife was at work, when she was called that I was in an operating room for craniology surgery to remove a bone from my skull to relieve pressure on my brain for the bleeding.

Once again, my wife and children found themselves at HCMC, waiting for news. The news was that the surgery went well, but staff didn't know anything except I was still in critical condition. Wish I could tell you about my month in HCMC, but I was in a medically induced coma, so that month does not register with me at all. I've been told I had multiple MRI or CAT scans, a tracheotomy, a feeding tube, as well as a session in the hyperbaric chamber. After being weaned from the drugs, in three days I started waking up from the coma.

As soon as I was awake, I was given a protective helmet and transferred to another hospital for cognitive therapy. During that second post-injury month, I needed to relearn everything our parents taught us before kindergarten. How to walk, eat, swallow, talk, get dressed, and use the bathroom—all the things we take for granted. It was during those therapy sessions that everyone, except me, knew my language skills were pretty much gone. My family tells me I talked like the Muppets' Swedish Chef. The hospital did remove my trach, and I was able to eat and drink, but needed a wheelchair as I lost a little bit of balance needed for walking.

For my third post-injury month, I was transferred to another hospital where I went to speech, occupational and physical therapy sessions twice a day, forty-five minutes per session. After a week, I gained my balance skills and didn't need a wheelchair, so physical therapy was only once a day. Occupational therapy was playing games on the computer or math quizzes. Speech therapy was perhaps the hardest thing I have ever done—trying to talk to be understood, trying to understand that others were saying, and trying to write. Part of my "pre-injury" job was teaching, and it was hard to believe that I couldn't communicate anymore.

In January 2004, because my physical skills were fine, I didn't need to live in a nursing home or rehabilitation center, so I was released from the hospital and went back home. I did however go to the Courage Kenny Rehabilitation Center to continue with speech and occupational therapy. In February 2004, I went back to HCMC for my final surgery to place my missing bone back on my skull. At the end of May 2004, I passed my driver's assessment and started driving again. That also meant I could try to go back to my "pre-injury" job. Because of therapy sessions, I couldn't work full-time, so I started with 8 hours a week, working up to 12 hours, 18 hours, and 22 hours. Not being able to work full-time was actually perfect because trying to fit in both therapy and work wore me out—I just couldn't do it. Fortunately, the company I work for gave me the time I needed. I can't thank them enough, as it seems I'm one of the few who hasn't lost their pre-injury profession. In October 2004, I did go back to work full-time as my therapists, my wife and I decided that work was the most important thing I could do to continue my healing and recovery process.

In 2010, things changed for the good. I was doing well, but the main side effects of my brain injury were short-term memory and aphasia (language).

To help with my short-term memory loss, I thought maybe a new hobby would help. To find out, I bought a mandolin, an instrument I never played before. This meant I needed to learn how to tune it, finger and strum chords, how to place my fingers on frets to play notes, how to pick those notes into a song, and most importantly how to remember that song an hour later, a day later, or a month later. Finding a new hobby is one of the best things I did after my injury as my short-term memory is much better.

Aphasia is the ability to know the word in your brain, and then be able to say it. Many times, instead of saying the correct word, my brain lets me say something else. For example, I was trying to say, "Give me the shampoo," but instead I said, "Give me the soup." Well, they both started with the letter S, but it's better to wash your hair with shampoo. To help with that, I talk to myself, read out loud, sing to myself (softly if in public), and talk back to the TV news reporters. I try to talk whenever I can.

I heard about the Minnesota Brain Injury Alliance, and took one of their classes. I also heard that Courage Kenny had a brain injury support group, and started attending their meetings. Going there really got me thinking. I was pretty sure that I was not the only person who survived a traumatic brain injury, but I had never met other survivors. I had never heard their stories, and never heard their tips or techniques for dealing with our "new" world. This support group helped me, and I decided that perhaps I could help other "new" survivors trying to navigate into a world they never expected to live. Yes, I wanted to give back for all the help and encouragement that my family, friends, co-workers, neighbors, and the volunteers who helped me and my family, gave during my first year. But, as the phase says, now I also wanted "to pay forward."

So, to do that, I became a member of Minnesota Brain Injury Alliance speaker bureau, and I became a facilitator for the Courage Kenny Brain Injury Support. I follow and post on brain injury online forums. I make my voice heard.

We don't have wear our injury as a badge, but we should never hide it. If you're asked to do something that you can't, because of the injury, tell them: *I didn't break my arm; I broke my brain. No, I'm not faking it, there's too much noise here.*

Even though a brain injury can happen to anyone, at any time, under any circumstance, many people think brain injuries only happens to soldiers because a bomb blast or to people after a violent attack. We survivors need to speak and make our voices heard. We need to be available to inform the general public what a brain injury is, and tell others that a brain injury doesn't just happen to one person, *it happens to their whole family.*

Doctors tell us that recovery is a two-year process, and that we will plateau. Doctors are wrong. As long as we never give up and keep trying, our recovery never stops.

Born in 1950, Ric lives in the Minnesota Twin Cities area and is a TBI survivor from October 2003. He is also a husband, father, and veteran. He's had many occupations including: commercial photographer, photography instructor, computer software teacher, website developer.

Chapter Sixty-Nine
An Incredibly Unexpected New Direction

Rick Smith
Madison, Wisconsin

For almost forty years my brain was the center of my world. Identified as "gifted and talented" at a very early age, I excelled at music, art, athletics, and academics. With the talent and ability to do anything and be anything I wanted, my brain became my identity, my playground, my sanctuary, and my most prized possession.

Music was my true passion, but economic pragmatism led me to the creative and analytical challenges of product design, where I also excelled. On any given day, you'll likely come across several of my designs, many of which were award-winning. Although my design work can be seen everywhere from football games to motorcycles to hospitals, my most memorable work is the International Design Excellence Award-winning tennis racket design used by Serena and Venus Williams to win the Australian Open and Wimbledon in 2005, respectively.

I was at the top of my game, including training to run a sub-3-hour Boston Marathon, when a chain-reaction car crash changed everything. In less than a second, the brain I cherished and worked a lifetime to create was irreparably damaged. My identity, my playground, my sanctuary, and my prized possession—were all gone. In their place a nightmare of medical neglect, insurance abandonment, financial devastation and legal roadblocks, not to mention never-before issues of thinking problems, neurochemical imbalances, and mental health issues all became my new daily reality.

It would take over a year for my own doctors and health insurer to begin to take my problems seriously. Fifteen months after the car crash, a forensic diffusion tensor imaging MRI would reveal widespread damage to several white matter tracts that connect different parts of my brain, and neuropsychological testing would reveal a drop of 17 IQ points. All the while this is happening, I am struggling with the hell that has become my life, and trying to figure out who am I, and where I go from here.

About that time, news broke of Suzy Favor Hamilton's double-life as a Las Vegas escort. In an instant her pristine image as a former American middle distance runner and three time Olympian was gone forever. Through the most unlikely of mental health-related circumstances, I knew exactly the loss of self as well as the immediate suicide threat that she was facing. I also knew if there was anything I could do to help her keep going, I'd never be able to forgive myself if I didn't act.

Suzy Favor Hamilton's ordeal, which ultimately led to her later being diagnosed with bipolar disorder, would end up shaping much of my recovery—giving me a sense of purpose, inspiring new possibilities, and providing examples of treatment paths. I would end up connecting with Suzy, and her kindness kept me from becoming a suicide statistic on more than one occasion. Her example and inspiration ultimately lead me to find a new identity and become Team USA duathlete, twice being the top USA finisher in my category at the ITU Duathlon World Championships.

Along the way, in addition to running the terrorist-bombed 2013 Boston Marathon, I realized the unique opportunity I have to help others overcome similar challenges, to help reshape the conversations surrounding traumatic brain injury and mental illness, and to help bring organization to the disjointed explosion of efforts to end stigma.

I wish I could say my story ended there, but TBI's many challenges are lifelong, and with those challenges come setbacks. Sadly, the past year and a half has been filled with the deepest, darkest and most prolonged depression of my life. Despite trying several additional medications during that time no real progress was made. Thankfully though, in yet another strange twist of fate, I'm just now beginning to find my footing due to, of all things, a medication for bipolar disorder.

Now the rebuilding process begins anew. Whether the road back leads to where I left off, or in an entirely new direction I go forward knowing that, with perseverance in the never ending fight that is TBI, unexpected and amazing things truly are possible.

Rick Smith is a former product design professional with numerous patents and design awards to his credit. Following a career-ending brain injury Rick found new direction as a three time Team USA qualifier in duathlon and has twice competed for Team USA at the ITU Duathlon World Championships. Today Rick continues to reshape himself and his life in the wake of his brain injury.

Chapter Seventy
The Concussion That Changed My Life

Robert Lee
Seattle, Washington

As a few of my friends know, I had a severe brain injury over 5½ years ago in June 2010 when I got rear-ended by a loaded cargo van doing 65 mph on I-5 going through downtown Seattle just before lunch. It crushed the front and back of my minivan, and I walked away with severe whiplash, as well spine and hip injuries.

What I didn't know *until 7 months later* on January 2011 was that I'd also sustained a serious brain injury. For me, the symptoms didn't really manifest completely until early the next year. I'd find myself walking into another room, and then wondering what I was doing there.

Since then I've learned so much from other people in the many brain injury support groups I continue to stumble across everywhere: social networks, local support meet-ups and national organizations. I certainly had no idea so much support was available.

But after months and months of chiropractic care, massage and physical therapy, the insurance companies were already preparing to cut me off from further treatment. So you can imagine their response when I tried to tell them I needed to go in for neurological testing: "Well, a neurologist visit will probably run around $3,000. If you decide to go to one, you can send us the bill. We might pay it, we might not."

I still remember sitting down to a Saturday evening dinner in Las Vegas with some of our guests and speakers at the end of another annual Football Veterans Conferences I organized. We'd just had two full days of speakers discussing a range of topics (including the ongoing lawsuits and concussions) with the retired football players attending the conference. I was describing my collision as part of our dinner conversation when Dr. Barry Sears leaned over and asked me, "Robert, do you have any idea how fast you need to be going in order to sustain a serious brain injury?"

I made what I thought was an educated guess: "Maybe around 25–30 miles-an-hour?"

Barry smiled at me and replied, "They've known for years that even with a 9-mile-an-hour impact, you can get a severe concussion!"

This one fact alone gets my blood boiling enough to wonder why a class action "What-did-you-know-and-when-did-you-know-it?" lawsuit hasn't ever been filed against the insurance companies? A day after my own collision, an appraiser looked at my vehicle and immediately told me to take it in to a professional auto body shop for a full appraisal on how much damage had been done—and they got me into a rental car. They knew that my vehicle had been rear-ended by a loaded cargo van on the freeway doing over 60 mph. But the customer, the person who actually pays the insurance policy? Unless you complain of physical injuries, the insurance company is never going to suggest you go to a doctor and certainly not a neurologist.

NOTE: I discovered that in many European countries, a neurologist is often sent out to the scene of an accident when it's likely people may have sustained brain injuries.

I was fortunate that we had been exploring hyperbaric oxygen therapy (HBOT) at some of the earlier conferences for retired football players. Some of those people mentioned that a small national trial was still recruiting football players and other brain injury victims as part of a trial to validate the use of hyperbarics in healing some of the effects of concussions. As luck would have it, there was a clinic where I lived that was part of this trial, so I managed to get in for testing to see if I qualified. This is how my friend and associate, Xavier, and I first met. He was the Research Director and managed the testing for the clinic. I managed to get in later that spring of 2011 and made my way through over two hours of testing on a computer terminal (ANAM tests).

Once I completed the testing, I waited for my scores to be tallied and reviewed. A short while later, Xavier walked in and said,

"Congratulations! You qualify for the trial!"

"Does that mean *I failed the test?*" I asked.

"Sorry, I can't tell you that right now, Robert,"

My sessions didn't even start until after Labor Day that fall in 2011, 15 months after my accident. I spent 8 weeks of 1-hour sessions in a chamber 5 days a week for a total of 40 hours under 1½ atmospheres pressure breathing pure oxygen. Midway through my hyperbaric treatment, I was tested again and my scores were already improving. At the end of the 8-week treatment, my new cognitive scores were once again normal to above normal like they probably were before my accident. And they held that way when I was tested again once 6 months and then 12 months after the sessions.

But I hadn't been tested since then until I went through a similar round of tests over 4 years later at the Amen Clinic prior to my scan. You can take a guess at what my cognitive scores looked like by then. Most of the scores were below normal once again, showing my earlier decline a few years after my oxygen therapy.

So after years of sending retired NFL football players to the Amen Clinic for Dr. Amen's groundbreaking study of 100+ players' brains over 5 years ago, it was finally time to get myself in there to find out *what was going on in my own head.* I even recall envying these players for finally having access to such a great resource, albeit really late for many of these men that the NFL chose to completely ignore.

It's been a strange journey, making my way through some subtle and more often not-so-subtle changes both in my mind and in the life around me. What surprises me in this day and age is how our awareness of brain injuries is so random, and often confusing.

- You have *the NFL* still trying to do their spin on downplaying the long-term effects of multiple hits over the years of playing football, all while trying to show that they care.
- Then you have *insurance actuaries* with decades of statistics and information that they continue to withhold, while putting more concern in the condition of your vehicle than worrying about their paying customers who were riding in that vehicle.
- And you have *doctors* who look at all your physical symptoms while mostly ignoring any possibility of brain injuries.

As I keep telling everyone I talk to about brain injuries, *it seems the more we learn, the less we know.*

I've also found it very difficult to open up and write about something that's so deeply personal. I can only imagine how hard it must be for others who have had even more severe brain injuries (especially so many of my football friends). It's why it took me so long to finally sit down and finish this article about my concussion. But I'm hoping to keep sharing what I learn through my journey, as well as the stories that others have so openly shared with me. I want to encourage everyone to share their personal experiences and stories so we can all learn about something that has now reached epidemic proportions in our society.

Robert Lee is a career entrepreneur from Seattle whose diverse background encompasses computer programming and hardware design, marketing consulting, advertising and electronic payment systems. As the founder and chief strategist behind successful businesses in both the U.S. and Canada, he and his companies have received national media exposure over the years. Robert has been working as an advocate for retired NFL football players for over 8 years, and his work led him to the study of brain injuries.

Chapter Seventy-One
My Life's Journey

Robyn Alexander
Plymouth, Minnesota

Life is defined as the time from birth to death. We think of life as a long tour or journey through time.

I remember when I was young, my folks would show us home movies—that's what they were in the old days, not videos or DVDs. It sure was neat to see ourselves as we were, to see how we've grown and changed. It seems the video camera is a machine to record our journey through life. Of course we mostly catch the highlights, and usually only the good ones. But when we look back, the whole journey comes into focus, more like the humanistic "Lost in Space" show was. We have our own video show running all the time, and each person views his or her show differently, and even is influenced by the person's mood at the moment of presentation.

The other day I noticed a gray hair, which got me wondering what the next part of my life's journey will be like. It's been a roundabout journey so far. I was born, crawled around, learned to walk, romped about, swam, jogged 10ks, skied, wind-surfed and even skydived when I was a dare devil. All this happened in high school. Then I journeyed on to college where I studied Aerospace Engineering in Florida and finished up at the University of Minnesota. Next I joined the U.S. Air Force and was stationed at Edwards Air Force Base in California with future plans to work at NASA as a Mission Specialist—but that changed September 11, 1985.

I was hit by a semi-truck on base, and was in a coma for 6 weeks, and then my journey began all over again.

When I woke up six weeks later, I had to learn to walk, talk and think all over again. I even went through the "terrible twos," but I was 23-years-old, so I got really terrible.

I moved on, through the so-called teenager stage, where I started doing drugs—anti-seizure drugs! Everyone thought at first I was just being a "moody teenager," until they noticed familiar, irregular actions.

I went through a period where my doctors had *me* experimenting with new drugs. The drugs would even make me feel high at times. I got toxic once or twice. They tell me that my boyfriend was reading from the Torah in the synagogue while I was in the congregation, and I wouldn't stop giggling and laughing.

I think I'm finally growing up (again). I'm getting more okay with doing things wrong, and accepting others telling that I've done things wrong. In fact, I welcome hearing people's feelings about things, and I think of better ways to do things rather than finding a way to "attack" them.

On this new path in my journey, I've learned to write poetry, with or without rhyming, and I'm also journaling. Through this combination, I've found myself writing cards, and when I remember little things about a person, I add that to make the card more personal. I enjoy doing this, and those receiving my cards tell me they enjoy it as well.

My independent living workers have helped me develop daily living charts, needed because of my short-term memory loss. This helps restore my confidence, making independent living practical: Weekly, monthly, half a year, and yearly.

With my memory and reasoning loss, I find staying involved with other people gives meaning to my life. I can do this by involvement in Wilderness Inquiry, Brain Injury Group (BIG), different writers groups, and activities with others with disabilities. The transportation services I had used then help greatly, like buses and Metro Mobility for evening meetings, or when multiple bus routes are too detailed for me to follow.

I still have my visual memory, and that can help me by my writing things down because I can pull it out by seeing it in my mind. I've discovered rhyming helps me remember things, and found positive rhymes are essential to my wellbeing. I've learned it helps if it arouses an emotion in me—which is why the negatives are so easy to remember. I've learned to use the positives so I work hard at seeing the good in life. This can be wonderful in turning me around when I have problems, especially with people being impatient with me since my disability is invisible to those who don't know me well.

Singing songs can help me remember, too, another emotion-arousal technique. Exercising has helped greatly in my singing, and I've turned to songs to help alter my moods. When someone says to you that you can't sing, remember that *everyone can sing*. Singing really helps folks feel good, so next time you're feeling goofy, let it out!

FEELING GOOFY – LA DI DA, DA, DA, DA. FEELING GOOFY!

Robyn has lived in Minnesota since she was 13. Since her brain injury in 1985, she has been dedicated to educating the public about brain injuries and the importance of having a current health directive. She is on complete Social Security Disability, and received her treatment from the military. In her free time she enjoys time spent with family and friends.

Chapter Seventy-Two
Expect Miracles

Robyn Block
St. Clair, Minnesota

I was on a skiing trip in northern Minnesota on April 2, 2013. I was excited to be on vacation, and was ready to ski! Since I had skied about 10 times in my life, I decided I was ready for the Olympics. We were waiting for our room to be available, and thought we'd take one run down the hill.

That's where it started and ended for me. My friend held my hand going down the first part until we got to a section where I said, "I can do it the rest of the way." Little did I know, I couldn't. I started on my own and must have realized I was going too fast. I got out of control and ran into a tree, and this flung me over and cracked my head on a rock.

First I was sent by ambulance to a small hospital where the medi-vac chopper was called. Once at a major hospital, they couldn't stop the bleeding. They had to remove the left side of my skull for three months due to the swelling. My dad arrived at the hospital, not knowing what happened. When he finally found the waiting room, the surgeon came out and told my dad to make arrangements because he wasn't sure I'd make it through the night. He expressed they were surprised I even made it through the surgery.

I went into coma and spent another two weeks in ICU. I was responding to pain stimulus, which the doctors said was good. They did a CT scan on day two or three, and that's when they found signs of damage to my brain stem and a possible stroke. My lungs were bruised, and I had a small injury on my liver. They had to tie down my left side as I was trying to pull out the tubes, which is normal. I had fluid on my lungs, which they said was pneumonia.

At this point, the doctors were still unsure.

They did start to cut down my sedation, but they had to increase it again as it took a lot out of me to try and breath on my own. When I awoke after eleven days in a coma, I couldn't understand why I was in the hospital and what happened. I just wanted to go home.

Then I spent one day in step down from ICU and did inpatient rehab for 20 days. I was then released to go back home and do outpatient rehab for an additional 8 weeks.

- July 2, 2013 they put my skull flap back in.
- August 2014 I began speaking to college classes and other groups about my injury and how important a health care directive is.
- April 2, 2014 I was allowed to cut down; then go off of my seizure meds.

On April 11, 2014, I had two grand mal seizures. I knew something wasn't right that day. My then-boyfriend got me into the truck—where I had a minute-and-half seizure on the way to the hospital. He called to get a sheriff to lead him, and they couldn't so he made them aware he was driving fast and wasn't stopping until he got me to the hospital.

Within all my headaches and head pains It was getting harder to wash and brush my hair in certain spots. I realized something wasn't right. I went to the doctor who discovered the screws were starting to pop out. I then met with my original surgeon, and he told me he couldn't believe how far I've come. *He said I am truly a miracle.* First they thought I'd die, then be paralyzed, etc. When we talked about the screws, he told me to wait as long as I can, because it's very dangerous to replace my skull part. Right now I have my original, if that changes we have to do a silicon or plate in there.

Still to this day I can't work. I suffer with my concentration and headaches. However I stay positive, and try to teach others to stay positive!

I want to share, from my experience, *why having a health care directive is so important*!

My parents divorced, which tore up our family. I was close with my dad but not with my mom, so everyone knew I'd want him in charge. However I did not have a directive, nothing in writing. I was 28 and didn't even know about them, but wish I did. During this process, a lot was going on—like them not knowing if I was going to live, going to walk, and going to know who people even were.

If I had a health care directive, everyone including doctors, would know who and what I wanted. Please consider one. A health care directive is a written document that informs others of your wishes about your health care. It allows you to name a person ("agent") to decide for you if you are unable to decide. It also allows you to name an agent if you want someone else to decide for you.

Check if you state has one because I know Minnesota does. Health Care Directives - Minnesota Dept. of Health www.health.state.mn.us/divs/fpc/profinfo/advdir.htm

Robyn is a native of St. Clair, Minnesota. Since her brain injury in 2013 she has been dedicated to educating the public about brain injuries and the importance of a health directive. In her free time, she enjoys time spent with family and friends.

Chapter Seventy-Three
My Many Miracles

Sarana Spokes
Gold Coast, Australia

It was Saturday, September 4, 2010. I was 41-years-old, enjoying a day like any other day living on the Gold Coast in Australia.

I had a few girlfriends over that afternoon. My husband had gone to bed early. Later in the evening after I watched a movie, I walked downstairs. At the bottom, I felt sick and collapsed on the floor, and began to vomit.

It's 4 a.m. the next morning, and a med-call (after-hours home care) doctor has found me near the front door. He's standing over me saying, "You need to go to hospital now."

From that moment, I don't really remember what happened. In fact I don't even remember phoning the med-call doctor—a call that saved my life.

I woke my husband, Ben, saying, "There's a doctor here. You need to take me to hospital." The doctor had written a note: Right eye 3rd nerve palsy.

Ben jumped out of bed, and we drove to the hospital, FAST. They rushed me in and did an MRI. I had a ruptured brain aneurysm with bleeding on the brain. Ben was told about my "odds," that 'if' I survive and then get through surgery, I will most likely go home with some type of disability. Ben called our daughter and other family.

After five hours of surgery where endovascular coils were put in, the operation was a success. However we were warned about vasospasms—spasm causing closure of vessels/arteries, like having a stroke—that can occur after surgery. After a week in ICU, they moved me to a ward, and that night I had a vasospasm and was rushed back to ICU. A week later, I had another vasospasm. Ben and our daughter were with me day and night.

Taking my first shower, I reached for the towel, and realized, "I can't feel my hand." Another vasospasm, and this was a bad one. Ben called for help, and nurses and doctors came running. Now back in bed, drips/fluids were trying to force open my vessels/arteries to save my life.

My face was drooping. I had lost feeling in my body, lost my sight and speech. Three hours later I began to regain some feeling, sight and speech—avoiding the last resort of a far-more-serious brain operation.

After three weeks in ICU, and another week in a ward, I was going home. My only visible disability was that my right eyelid was permanently closed like it was asleep, and my eyeball was stuck looking outwards.

Recovery was slow at the start. I was in bed most days, with painful headaches, stuttering speech, and no sight in my right eye.

Each morning I would be grateful for that day, grab my eyelid, pull it open and try to blink, but it would close. I continued this routine every day for three months. Then the miracle happened, the lid opened a tiny bit. Six months later my eye opened fully. It took a while for my eye to regain sight. Lots of tests were done. I have double vision in my right eye, and it is permanently dilated, which I will have for life. Light affects me, but I'm getting used to it.

After three months, I went to my neurosurgeon for my check up. Everything looked like it was going reasonably well. I told the doctor I wanted to go back to work one day a week. The doctor said it was way too soon. I was determined, so he wrote me the necessary certificate.

Ben and our daughter said, "No." They were so worried something was going to happen to me, but I wasn't. I went back to work one day a week as a Childcare Director. The day before I would rest all day in bed.

I was so excited to work, even though I would still have headaches and my memory was bad. After working, the next day I would be in bed. But it was worth it. I felt normal. This was very hard for my family and friends as they were very concerned for my well being as I continued to push myself.

I did regular physio rehab, and other treatments that would help me. The next two years I was still slowly recovering—dealing with headaches, stuttering, noise and light affected me, left side numbness, double vision, and tremors.

I was happy to wake up each day. I wanted nothing more than to enjoy life and not live in fear. And that's what I tried to do.

I was positive and got on with life, but there were times when I put up a front, and because my injury was internal, people wouldn't realize how hard some situations were for me. I often lied about how I was feeling, but many times there was no way I could hide it.

Explaining that I wanted to feel "normal," and being honest with my family and friends, helped them understand why I would push myself. However it didn't make it any easier for them as I repeatedly pushed myself to the limits, in order to feel "normal."

After lots of MRIs and CT scans, I went for my two-year check up. When I received the results—another aneurysm—I began to cry. When I came in for my second operation, I was first up. I wasn't scared or nervous; I was really relaxed. A nurse came in and said, "We've had three emergencies, and the ICU is full." They were sending me home with no operation. I balled my eyes out.

Two weeks later, January 2013, it was my turn again. When I asked a nurse if I would get to see the surgeon, she said, "We usually have you under before he arrives."

"I would love to meet him, he saved my life." She had a tear, and so did I.

The surgeon came in and said "Hi." I smiled and with tears rolling down my face, I thanked him for saving my life two years earlier.

He said, "You're welcome. You ready for this?"

"With you as my surgeon, I sure am."

"Okay, lets go."

The operation went well. My surgeon put in a "pipeline flow diverting stent" below both aneurysms. After a week in ICU and then two weeks in a ward, I was going home again.

Three months later I returned to doing childcare, driving myself to work when I was able. Some days it was a huge struggle, and I could not make it through the entire day. With all the love and support from the woman I job shared with, my manager and staff, I got through it.

After a few years back at work, I had to face that it was taking its toll on my health. I was still having migraines, tremors, along with bouts of anxiety—later diagnosed as PTSD from my traumatic experience. I resigned, which made me very upset, but I realised it was the best thing for me.

This journey has been so very hard. By necessity I've had to dramatically slow my pace of life. I can rarely drive, and when I do, I stay very close to home. In a way, I've lost some independence.

It's also been hard for my husband, our daughter, and family. Our 22-year-old daughter has put her life on hold for me. I'm so blessed to have their love and support.

Now September 2016—six years later, what really matters? For me, it's family and friends. We always remember we are together. We smile, laugh, love, and feel grateful.

Most people don't understand TBI because you can't always see it. It can affect different people in so many different ways. If you're reading this and you've had a TBI, I wish you love and the best for your future. Have hope.

If you happen to know or meet anyone with a TBI, be patient and make time for them. Your love and support matters.

Sarana Spokes worked in the child care Industry for 27 years. After a ruptured aneurysm to the brain, and having a second brain operation, she had to resign, and now is trying to spend quality time with family and friends.

Chapter Seventy-Four
The Invisible Years

Sera Rathbun
Pullman, Washington

Turning 16 is always a highlight for Americans. It's the day when we finally have the opportunity to gain our coveted driving license, and with it, more independence and perhaps a shiny new car. Living in a rural area, my parents were quite pleased when my brother, and later, I got our driving licenses because it meant a reprieve from the long hours of taxi services that they were providing to us on top of their already-extensive commuting hours for their jobs. We each had the same "starter car"—Dad's green 1973 Porsche 914. We drove this car up and down our driveway in the months and weeks preceding the dawn of our 16th birthdays, when we could legally drive it out onto the highway. It was a great car, cute, semi-dependable, and the heater would start working after a couple hours of driving, and it was the car Dad was driving when he met Mom. We soon found out that it also was incredibly sturdy.

Six days after turning 16, on March 7, 2002, I was driving home from school in the dark. A semi-truck began tailgating me just outside of town, and then refused to pass when opportunity arose several times in the ensuing eight miles. Finding myself in a rather dire situation requiring a left turn to get home, and being unable to pull off to the right because the sudden decrease in speed would almost certainly be met with a collision, I chose to turn left onto a county road so that I could manage the turn at my speed. I signaled more than 1000 feet ahead of my turn, but I didn't realize that the semi was too close to me to see my signal. He was looking right over the top of my little Porsche and couldn't see my taillights.

I accelerated even faster to put some distance between us, and attempted the left turn at the Y onto the county road. At this exact moment, the semi driver decided that he would like to pass this pesky little Porsche in front of him, on a corner, right before a hill, and at an intersection. As soon as he pulled out to overtake me, he realized his mistake in judgment and tried to correct. He hit me in the exact center of my rear bumper with his momentum going one way, while mine was going the other. This is where the mid-engine design of the Porsche kept me from rolling (and kept the semi-truck from barging right into my car, which contained me) but instead I spun, at high speed. I watched the stop sign at the county road/highway intersection go by three times before I stopped right next to it. In my memory, I then turned off my car and got out. Though, later piecing the incident back together, about five minutes were unaccounted for, during which I was probably unconscious.

There had been no impact between my head and any part of the car, but my brain had moved around in my skull as a result of the intense forces that come with spinning at high speed, and diffuse brain damage had occurred. However, this was a time when the average medic or primary care physician did not think of head injuries, especially in "mild" circumstances. I had exited the car and was walking and talking, so I was taken to the hospital as a precautionary measure to check for a neck injury.

No one thought to investigate the condition of my brain. My brain started to swell and, four days later, I became very nauseated and lost my ability to walk and talk. Even then, as Mom searched for answers, no one thought to consider a closed-head injury.

Mom is a physical therapist, so that was one major thing I had going for me. She worked with me, and her friends and colleagues did the same. *Six years later*, after seeing at least eight different neurologists, it was finally diagnosed as a TBI, and rehab was offered. One wonders if the outcome would have been different had my brain injury been quickly diagnosed and treated, instead of being addressed after the supposed plateau of recovery, five years post-injury. Medical bills piled up throughout those years also, but a settlement was eventually reached that reimbursed our expenses. I have since added much more coverage to my car insurance, as the $10,000 included in my policy at the time didn't last very long into my recovery. Yes, the plateau of recovery is thought to have occurred five years post injury, but my injury wasn't even diagnosed until six years post-injury.

Another thing I had going for me, a bittersweet luck of the draw—I was young. Young brains can recover more fully, but they also face the reality that, if a full recovery isn't possible, the young brain has many years and many life experiences ahead that must be navigated through a TBI: college, marriage, work, old age. I know many of us feel unheard and unseen after we have gone through our rehab and adjusted to our new normal, but no one talks about the decades that follow, and the effects our TBI has on everyone who chooses to be a part of our lives. The doctors aren't involved anymore. The therapists have moved on to new patients. And, we learn that the new normal we've found in one stage of life can be turned completely upside down as we try to navigate the next stage.

Being fourteen years post-injury, and now at age thirty, I feel like *only in the last year* have I been able to gain more realistic long-term perspectives of life with a TBI. During this last March, Brain Injury Awareness month, I made it a priority to post on Facebook nearly every day about some specific struggles we long-termers are facing (these are public posts and can be found if you search my name). I do this in the hopes that awareness can be raised among the public at large, as well as perhaps those living with an undiagnosed TBI, that they might find some answers to their questions and seek help now with more confidence that they are not alone. I was surprised by the insistent encouragement I received from many to write a book to expand on these thoughts, so that is my task for this year.

It has taken me 14 years to not only come to some more specific conclusions about TBI-induced life challenges, but to gain the courage to speak out publicly. I think I am not alone in my experiences with doctors who diagnosed me with chronic and incurable psychosomatic disorders. I quote from the treatment notes of one, among many:
- Client's thought process was linear and logical except with regard to her physical difficulties.
- Client would be extremely irritating to supervisors or coworkers due to her insistence of a disability.
- Would client benefit from psychological help? No, the client is too entrenched and has had a lifetime of reinforcement.

Not only did they not spend enough time with me to make a correct diagnosis, they sent me home with no referral for further care or evaluation. If they truly believed that I had a psychological disorder, they could have at least sent me to a counselor or psychiatrist, instead of just sending me home to deal with things on my own—and hopefully *not commit suicide*. I eventually did see a counselor and a psychologist on my own accord, and they sent me back to a neurologist, stating that I had neurological symptoms that had been grossly overlooked.

Looking back, I am baffled by how many cracks I fell into, and could have stayed in, had it not been for Mom continuing to seek answers. I was not in a capable state to be my own advocate. Many TBI survivors find themselves without someone to fight for them. What becomes of those people?

I appreciate the advancement in concussion awareness that has come out of the NFL and other high-profile sports. I know that the advancement in awareness and treatment will eventually trickle down to us in the anonymous crowd. I am also thankful that it is changing the perception of a TBI to one on the level of any other injury, because it is simply another sports injury in this high-profile situation, as opposed to being something not understood, therefore not real, and therefore untreatable. More doctors and healthcare professionals are looking for TBIs, even when the impact has been relatively minor.

I appreciate these advancements, and they have given me courage to speak out and to be publicly labeled with a disability.

Sera lives in the beautiful Palouse area of Washington state with her husband and two dogs. She spends her time cycling, swimming, and learning languages, hoping to become a translator at some point in the future, as official employment is as yet too difficult to navigate. She also loves music and plays the violin.

Chapter Seventy-Five
Our Story of Poisoning — and of Grace

Shelley Taylor and Taylor Trammell
Grand Prairie, Texas

We had been without electricity for three days due to the weather, and earlier in the day we ran a generator out in the driveway/edge of our garage—we had the garage door open, windows in garage open, etc. The fire chief later told us that since it was so cold, with no wind, the gas probably just settled instead of blowing away, and then crept back into the house via the eaves.

Thirteen-year-old Taylor and I had gone to bed in our respective bedrooms. Later she told us that someone called her name, and when she tried to get up to see who it was, she shimmied up against her wall before collapsing at the edge of her bedroom. The thud of her falling woke me up. Charlie (her dad, and my then-husband) also heard this from the living room, and when he and I went to the hallway to see what it was, we found her lying lifeless facedown. We couldn't get her to respond, and Charlie sent me for the flashlight by my bed. On my way to the bedroom, I started feeling like something was not right with me either. I grabbed the flashlight, and started running back to the hall so I could let him know I wasn't okay. I knew if I collapsed in the bedroom he wouldn't know to come for me, and I had to get to him so he would know I was sick. The closer I got to them, the further away I felt like I was getting. Everything was spinning out of control. When I turned the corner to the hallway, I collapsed face first without any hands/arms to brace me, falling onto the metal flashlight, cutting my forehead to the bone.

Charlie had to search in the dark for the flashlight as it had rolled when I fell, and I told him I felt blood running down my face. Once he found the flashlight, he said he had to get me to the hospital. I said, "What is wrong with Taylor, doesn't she need to go?" Taylor meanwhile was in and out of consciousness. He was able to get her to wake up, and told her she had to get a towel to put on my head to help with the bleeding until help got there. My head began to pulse blood out of control. When she returned with the towel, she again became unconscious not far from me, and Charlie had to drag her over and prop her on top of me, against the wall as I was having convulsions and banging my face into the concrete floor. My eyes were rolling back in my head, and Charlie was yelling that "I wasn't going to die on him!"

Charlie called 911, and first to respond were the police. Immediately upon entering they looked for the lights, and Charlie told them we were without power. Using their flashlights, they saw my blood, bloody handprints on the hallway walls where I tried to stand up after I fell, and Charlie had blood on him. Right away they began accusing him of a crime, and he explained what had transpired. Shortly the fire department arrived, and luckily Charlie knew one of the firemen who came to his defense. The fire chief began asking what we had done earlier in the day to try to put some of the pieces together about what had happened.

When Charlie told of the generator use, the fire chief went directly to the truck to get the carbon monoxide detector. The truck was parked at the street, and within steps of entering our driveway, the detector began to "freak out" so much that the chief went back to the truck to recalibrate the devise because he did not believe the high readings. Once again, walking in the driveway up to our front door, the readings on the devise began to creep higher and higher. Upon reaching the door, the chief called for his crew to get Charlie, Taylor, and our dogs out and then exit our home. A couple of paramedics were left inside to get me stable enough for transport to the hospital. Once outside, they realized that Taylor had "started" this whole incident, and the firemen told Charlie they also wanted her checked out. I left by ambulance and Charlie and Taylor followed in his truck.

Several firemen stayed at our home to open windows and to watch our dogs for sickness, and make sure they were in a safe place before leaving. This was way beyond the call of duty. Once at Mansfield Methodist, the staff checked both my and Taylor's blood gases, which were "through the roof"; hers much higher than mine.

Mansfield Methodist was not prepared or skilled to handle emergencies such as ours, and they began preparing us to be transported to Dallas Methodist in an ambulance on icy roads. They needed to get us in the hyperbaric chamber. First my head had fifteen stitches, and I had to have a CT to make sure I was transportable. Off we went, Taylor and me in the ambulance, her sitting with oxygen on and me on a stretcher with oxygen on. Somewhere along the way my oxygen ran out, and the facemask adhered to my face, not a fun experience. The paramedics were wonderful. Upon arriving at Dallas Methodist, they began to explain the procedures for going into the hyperbaric chamber—all of this I am trying to comprehend while the carbon monoxide is still doing damage to my brain!

Sometime after our arrival, we learned that the family that had just been in the chamber all died, except the father. Not comforting! Taylor and I are both very claustrophobic, but we survived our approximate three-hour stay in the hyperbaric chamber. Taylor was such a trooper, as they had a very difficult time getting her to the depth that we needed to be to be successful. Two ambulance rides, one CT Scan, two blood gases, two hyperbaric chambers, fifteen stitches and one concussion later, WE SURVIVED! Nothing says "I love you" like a brain injury on Valentine's Day, February 14, 2010.

Afterwards my sister moved in for approximately a month. Physically I was trying to heal my head, but mentally I was left with a traumatic brain injury. I literally started over with kindergarten flashcards, looking at an apple but saying "library." Friends and family scooped Taylor and me up and helped us heal. My neurologist told me that people don't survive what we went through, and there really aren't patients like us. He said they really don't know how to treat me. Through his honesty, he became a great comforter as I struggled so with memory and cognitive skills. My short-term memory is horrible at times, and I've lost so many precious memories. Taylor and I have a saying when it comes to trying to remember things, we just look at each other and ask, "Did we have fun?" The one who remembers says to the other, "Yes, we had fun!" That's all that matters. But, to be alive is amazing—in whatever capacity. God is good; no, He's great, and His grace is unending!

The worse things I daily deal with are breathing, memory and balance, or lack thereof. Both Taylor and I struggle with this every day. I have fallen more times than I've stood, it seems, and I've forgotten more than I remember. I've had injuries that ranged from Band-Aids to orthopedics visits. Recovery continues every day for Taylor and me. Luckily her dyslexic brain is used to accommodating skills, and this continues to be her saving grace. She is young, and healing has come differently for her, but memory and migraines are her big battles.

Side note: When we arrived home from the hospital, I grabbed Taylor's forearms and said to her, "You know the voice that woke you up was not me or daddy?" Her response, "I KNOW MOM!" My faith is amazing! God's grace and mercy is incredible.

Taylor Trammell is the subject of the book "Living 'Lexi': A Walk in the Life of a Dyslexic." She is currently studying to become an American Sign Language Interpreter, graduating in May 2017. Taylor is a leader of Embrace Grace (a ministry for single pregnant girls), she's very creative and displays this through the lens of her camera.

Shelley Taylor is a therapeutic writer and published author of "Living 'Lexi': A Walk in the Life of a Dyslexic" and is currently writing "With My Last Breath I'd Say I Love You: When Your FAITH and HOPE Slip, GRACE Wins Every Time." Shelley is happily married to the man of her dreams, a mom of six, "Honey" to eight and a Certified School Risk Manager by day. Shelley is a leader of Embrace Grace (a ministry for single pregnant girls) and lives every day trying to help people heal through her written words. www.shelleytaylor.net

Chapter Seventy-Six
From a Dream to a Nightmare to Reality

Shelly Lorden
Hamburg, New York

On a cold January day in 2012, I stood there staring out the window. I was numb, painfully numb, and didn't feel anything. Yet I was semi aware of my dark and cold surroundings. I was standing close to a window and could feel the chill embrace me. I hugged myself tightly to get warm while random thoughts where flashing in my mind, but nothing came that I could grab and hold onto.

I could also hear sounds, but they were strange and unfamiliar ones—little bells and bleeps. I must be dreaming. I can smell some unknown odors, neither a good nor a bad smell, but nothing in my memory that indicated what it was.

As I continue to look out this window, I notice a beautiful house. Ohhh, it was purple, my favorite color. It had high peaks and beautifully ornate carved woodwork that was painted a contrast of a much lighter shade of purple. If I had seen this house yesterday, I would have had a lot more to say about it. I can be a chatty Cathy. But right now I couldn't even muster what that might have been. As I looked at this quiet, still house without a light on, it began to snow. I still didn't feel anything. Weird.

At first it was a very few light flakes, then bigger fluffier flakes, then ginormous flakes. As I was watching, I noticed that it wasn't just any old snow…it was Christmas snow! You know, the snow that glitters and sparkles, and makes the world seem so much more beautiful. It's the kind that causes a miracle, and maybe Santa Clause might be real. Most people hate snow, but not me.

These people would complain, complain, complain, and it felt like they were stomping on my heart. Anyway, I would think to myself, if you hate it so much, than just move south or go west. And some did. In the summer these people would go on about how it was too hot or too rainy, and again complain, complain, complain. I would say, "Hey this is Buffalo, the Miami of the North. We have the most beautiful sunsets in the entire world."

As for me, *I love snow*. When I learned that Eskimos have over fifty names for it, I started taking pictures and named the different kinds I see. My personal journal of snow, love it or hate it, I have a word or words for it. Crunchy snow, good packing snow, light fluffy snow, snow globe snow, slushy snow, crisp snow, heavy snow (which is difficult to shovel, so be careful)...oh the list goes on and on. My favorite is Christmas snow, and this is what I was looking at. Ever since I could remember, seeing this type is like going to church. God and I always seemed to have a meeting of the minds, or just a word (always different), but always an experience. Once when I was walking home, it started snowing Christmas snow, and I just stopped, put my arms up and started spinning. Christmas snow always had a presence of peace about it. That's what it was! It made me feel peaceful.

Oh, I just felt something that brought me back to where I was. I slowly turned and walked away from the cold window. I looked down and gazed upon my youngest daughter. I grabbed ahold of her hand. She is beautiful, with long silky blonde hair, hazel eyes and long eyelashes. She loves reading and arguing, doing laundry and stealing her sisters' clothes.

Suddenly I am aware of the bells and bleep sounds and smells again. Why was I unable to feel, and why don't I want to feel, or think? I cannot utter a word. I can only look around and observe this new world that I am in. The room is very sterile, yet I can see blood. I see order, yet also chaos. I turn my head sideways, as a dog does when it doesn't understand what you are saying. As I'm tilting my head sideways and looking baffled, I see a man's face lit up by a computer screen. What is he doing? Why is he so focused? My thoughts are broken by a nurse who begins to ask me questions. I have no recollection of what she said, but got the idea that she wanted me to try resting, and to know if I needed anything. No, I didn't feel as if I needed anything. So I let go of my daughter's hand and sat down. I could not escape these sounds.

I don't remember falling asleep. I woke up to many doctors and nurses talking and discussing things. Hmm, I was hearing my daughter's name mentioned more than once, which of course, increased my curiosity. I lifted the cover from my head. I had put it there to try to keep those sounds out of my mind. When they noticed that I was awake, a short Asian man approached me. He explained he was the Chief of Neurosurgery, and that he and his staff had to do surgery today. Why is he telling me this?

And bam! Memories instantly flooded my mind faster than lightning, and were hard to compute. It was like my brain rebooted and a million lines of reprograming where just scrolling in front of my face. It finally stopped. The phone was ringing at the time of night when you know that no one should be calling you. It was a sheriff's deputy, and I was to go to the hospital immediately. Confusion consumed me. I remember getting in my car and driving and being overcome with a sick feeling—and praying, please let everything be okay.

When I arrived, I was greeted by a doctor. I could see the look in her eyes—mother to mother. Something was not right. She explained that my beautiful daughter had been in a terrible car accident, and things were not looking good. My breathing became heavy. She ever so calmly tried to prepare me for the worst, which at this moment was organ donation, because they did not expect her to survive. My head went into a tailspin. She took me to a room where I could wait until I was able to see my daughter. As I walked into this room, it seemed to be spinning. I just stood there.

I wonder now, how many people are brought to this room? I think it is *one too many* that ever should have to be. But nonetheless, here I was now in this, room, spinning. I'm not sure how much time passed before I realized that almost everyone I knew and my daughter knew, were in the room with me. Still unable to speak, I can only observe what is going on around me. Now I see my other daughters enter the room, and I grab and hold them. Then I felt peace...yes, it is all going to be okay. They began to explain what happened and were revealing to me that it was bad, really bad. No! How? This is all a terrible dream. I grabbed ahold of my other daughters, not ever wanting to let go—and to be out of this room.

A memory flashed about spinning in the Christmas snow, and that thought was very comforting. How I wanted to cling onto that easiness of life. Everything changed in the blink of an eye—a glimpse of the present. Then reality, with its big hammer, loudly began hitting me over and over as reality began to set in.

My beautiful 13-year-old daughter had been in a horrific car accident.

When a nurse enters and escorts me down a long hallway, I felt as if I were floating. She brings me to a cold, dark room where I look upon my child as she lay motionless, clinging to life. All kinds of tubes were coming out of her. Now I can identify the sounds, it is those machines keeping her alive. And the smells where the undeniable scents of a hospital. That man on the computer was her nurse who was monitoring every detail of her new, frail state. A tear runs down my face, and I turn and look out the window.

Our lives will never be the same. Four and a half years later my daughter has 98 percent recovered physically, which is a miracle in itself. She had much to overcome, like learning to breathe, walk, talk and eat all over again. We now deal with the daily issues caused by her TBI.

She is currently attending a specialized school in hopes to get her high school diploma and resides with her mom.

Shelly is a mother of four beautiful children from Buffalo, New York. On a cold night in January, she received the "parents worst nightmare" call. Her youngest daughter was involved in a horrific car accident. This is Shelly's short story of the shock-filled first hours of being in the hospital with the realization of what has happened to her daughter.

Chapter Seventy-Seven
I'm Very Grateful

Shelly Millsap
Glendale, Arizona

Oh crap! That is the last thing that I remember thinking as I looked at the microwave clock and realized that I was running late for work. Now looking back, why was that so important? No one would care if I were 2 minutes, 5 minutes or even 3 hours late… I owned my own business and had no other employees. Why was it so important to me to be out of the door at a certain time each day? Why didn't I stand there in my kitchen and take one more sip out of my cup before hurrying off to work? Why didn't I turn left in the kitchen to throw my napkin away instead of going right? *"Why" is a powerful question, one I can't live my life wondering.*

So many things could easily have changed the outcome of that day—just one step to the left, one more sip out of my cup, or just one more minute of standing still and not worrying about being late for my day.

January 17, 2013—1,673 days, 4 hours and 4 minutes ago at this writing, my life changed forever. I was standing in my kitchen drinking some juice, about to leave for work. I looked at the microwave clock and realized that I was running behind. I had a long list of work duties to accomplish that day, so I needed to hurry up. I put my cup in the sink, and that is when I heard a noise and turned my head. I thought, "Why am I falling to the ground?" as I put my hand up to my face. I closed my eyes. When I opened them again, I looked and didn't understand why blood was splattered around and dripping off of me. Why did my face feel numb? Why was I on the floor?

Nothing made sense. I put a towel up to my face. I tried to stand up, but I couldn't. I had very little energy. Looking at the microwave clock, the time made little sense. How had 20 minutes passed by?

Why was my face starting to pound from pain? Why was there blood continuing to drip down my face? I sat there for a few minutes until somewhere inside, I found the strength to pull myself up and went to a mirror. Panic struck. What had happened? Why was my nose no longer straight on my face? Why was my face so swollen and bleeding? I tried getting my phone to take a photo. Not sure why I thought that was important at the moment. I tried taking the photo, but I was trembling so much that the phone fell to the floor. I knew I needed help, so I called my husband at work. I'm not sure what I said, but told him I had been hurt. I snapped and sent him a photo of my gruesome face before I moved to the couch.

My husband called back once he saw the photo I had sent him. I told him that I needed to get some medical help, but I didn't know what to do. We were relatively new to the area, and I didn't know anyone, so I decided to drive myself. Looking back, that was insane. I went out to the car and found that it was frozen over with ice. We were living in Idaho at the time, and January is always full of ice and snow. Once inside the car, I couldn't see out of the windshield because of all the ice. I turned on the defrost, but decided I couldn't wait any longer, and started to drive once a tiny, four-inch spot was defrosted and open on the windshield. Driving with one hand, because the other was holding the towel on my face for the blood, I drove myself down the street. The entire car was so frozen over I had to open the door at intersections to see if the traffic was clear.

Luckily, about a mile away, I pulled into the parking lot of a clinic. When I walked in and asked if they could help, they looked at me in disbelief, and immediately took me into the backroom. My husband was contacted and told that they were transporting me to the hospital.

Putting all of the pieces together, this is what had happened. A few weeks prior to January 17, 2013, I had made a bottle of homemade ginger ale from a recipe on the internet. After it sat in the refrigerator for two weeks taking up valuable space, and no one drinking it, I took it out and put it on the counter next to the sink. Being super busy with work, I never poured it out. It sat on the counter fermenting enough to become a bomb ready to detonate, and I would be its eventual target.

I was running late for work when I passed by this ticking time bomb, as it exploded in my face. I was knocked unconscious for 20 minutes.

The first few days after my accident, I was fine, but had bruises all over, and a broken nose. I was lucky. I even went to work the very next day to try and make up for the work I had missed the day prior. But after going to the doctor a few days later for a follow up, I was told that a concussion is a serious thing, and I needed to be at home doing absolutely nothing…no TV, no computer, no reading, no work…NOTHING! I called my clients and said that I'd be taking a few days off due to my accident, but promised them that I'd be up and running after the weekend. I did as was told, and was the most bored person in the entire world.

Little did I know at the time—that would be my last day of work.

A few days later, things started to change. Normal, everyday things started to become difficult. Words didn't come to mind, and I also struggled to form words. I started having problems walking, and eventually started dragging my right leg behind me when I walked. After many tests and many doctors' visits over the next few weeks, they didn't find anything other than a TBI. I was lucky. The doctor said that I had suffered from an Axonal brain injury, and 90 percent of people don't wake up from this type of trauma. After months of speech therapy and physical therapy, I was back to my old self—at least on the outside. The TBI had left me with injuries on the inside that I am still trying to deal with 3½ years later.

But I feel grateful and lucky.

I feel grateful and lucky because I am alive. I feel grateful and lucky because I get to spend more time with my children and husband. I feel grateful and lucky that my outer shell isn't disfigured. I feel grateful and lucky that maybe I can touch someone else's life due to my experiences, and help them. I am not who I was before. I can no longer be in loud spaces or around a lot of people. I still suffer from

PTSD and cry every Fourth of July due to the noise from fireworks exploding. But I choose to live. I choose to be grateful and happy. I choose every single day not to have a pity party. I choose every day to eat a piece of chocolate because that makes me happy (and a few pounds heavier).

Since my accident, I have not been able to work. I spend my days trying to relearn the things that I have forgotten how to do because of my accident. I'm lucky. My brain is allowing me to relearn things with a lot of hard work and repetition. I will never be who I was before. How could I be? I have gone through a life-altering ordeal, and it has changed me forever. I choose to believe that it has changed me for the better. I still need a lot of help, and have a long way to go, but I am a persistent little thorn in the back of my TBI.

I'm not ever going to give up trying. I know that I have new limitations and a new "normal," as the doctors like to say. I just keep putting one foot in front of the other and keep trudging along my new path in life. I am forever grateful to the people and doctors that have helped me along the way, and most of all to my family. When I couldn't talk, they spoke for me. When I couldn't walk, they held me up. I am fortunate to have such a great husband and two compassionate sons. I know that their lives have also been forever changed due to the journey they have had to take with me. I know that this has made all of us more compassionate and caring people for everything.

This is my story. This is my new life, and I am a TBI survivor.

Shelly Millsap is a mother to two sons, and has been married to her husband, Bob, for 22 years. She has been a fourth grade teacher, the owner of The Sweet Bakerista, and a volunteer in her church and community. She enjoys being creative by baking, crocheting, and sewing. She tries to always focus on helping others who are in need.

Chapter Seventy-Eight
Life is a Lesson

Stanley H. Wotring, Jr.
Lynn, Massachusetts

October 7, 1981 was a morning like any other morning in my hectic college life. Living with my grandmother while I attended school made the rigors of a busy schedule not so tough. It required a six-mile commute along the curvy mountain roads to West Virginia Wesleyan College, but I had been given an SUV for high school graduation so I was prepared.

They said I swerved to miss a dog or a kid chasing a dog. I don't remember, and no one came forth to claim responsibility. It doesn't matter; the result was still the same. My car went over a 50-foot embankment, rolling over and over, causing me to be thrown from it like a projectile, and my forward movement was stopped by a fallen log.

Although I was fortunate enough to have no broken bones and only a small cut on the left side of my head, I would not regain consciousness for eleven more days. Back then, med-flights were unheard of, at least in such a rural area. I was not expected to survive the ambulance ride from the local hospital to the University hospital, but I did.

This *would not be* the last time I would defy a pessimistic prognosis.

Not understanding why I had not regained consciousness yet, the doctors did not hold out much hope that I would be more than in a vegetative state. Still such pessimism did not dampen my family's spirit as they took turns being by my side to make sure I was never alone. In the background, my favorite music was constantly played to give me some life preserver of my past reality to cling to. Doctors had tried to convince my parents to transfer me to a nursing home, but they stubbornly refused, insisting that when I left the hospital, I would be going home.

So after about a month in the hospital, I was sent home. I still was not speaking yet, and was oblivious to my condition. In fact I have no recollection of my hospital stay, or even anything up until the time I started speaking a week later. When that happened, I truly regained full consciousness and was able to take charge of my recovery. Take charge I did. I spent countless hours exercising with Dad, Mother and brother by my side, encouraging my every effort.

I also signed up for outreach college courses through the mail before I could walk again. Although they negatively impacted my G.P.A., I feel confident they were crucial to my recovery and allowed me to return to college full time the following August. I even got an "A" in Organic Chemistry my first semester back. Chemistry had always been my strong point, winning the Freshman Chemistry Award the year before.

However my previous plans for med school were not going to come to fruition. While my professors did not doubt my academic abilities, they were hesitant for me to pursue a career in the medical field for fear of my social acceptance in that community. Instead they tried to steer me into seeking a Ph.D. in Biochemistry. I rebelled at that advice and got a degree in psychology to get out of the academic environment as soon as I could, graduating in 1985 with a BA in psychology.

I've lived with the consequences of that decision ever since.

While I have not received the financial success I had once dreamed of, I have found that this slower life has given me new perspectives to be able to see riches all around me. I had a contract with a Hollywood production company that never panned out, but how many people can even say they had one. I've conducted a poetry workshop several years ago at the West Virginia Writers Conference (I didn't even like poetry at the time), and later moved to Massachusetts where I would retire from the Division of Developmental Services and raise beautiful brother and sister twins.

My life has been very difficult and challenging at times, yet I am thankful to have gained the experiences I have had because they have given me the perspective to appreciate what I have, and value the possibilities I can achieve. You cannot change the past, but you can learn from it.

On the way to Physics class at West Virginia Wesleyan College, Stanley swerved to miss a dog, went over a 50-foot embankment and spent eleven days in a coma back in 1981. Life's been a journey for him, but he's been lucky enough to graduate from college, retire from working for the State of Massachusetts, and raise beautiful twins. Now he spends his time thinking and writing.

Chapter Seventy-Nine
The Power of Never Giving Up

Stephanie M. Freeman
Rochelle, Georgia

I am a single mother and runner from the state of Georgia. And running isn't something that has so easily come to my life.

At the age of fourteen, I lived two months of my life in a coma on life support. This was from a brain injury I received in an automobile accident on June 4, 1993. I experienced a traumatic brain injury and lung injury, and was not expected to survive. However, with faith, strength and determination, I did pull through. I awoke to the realization that I was bound to a wheelchair and unable to walk. I was told I would be leaving that hospital a handicapped child because they had no hopes I'd ever walk again.

I recall that day in August so vividly in my mind. I woke up and knew who and where I was, and I have recalled that day every day since 1993. Sitting in front of a nurse's station with my head hanging down, I had spit rolling uncontrollably from my mouth. I slowly lifted up my head and glanced around me. That's when I discovered I was sitting in a wheelchair. I had no clue that I had been in a coma two months, and no clue I had a brain injury. I remember asking myself as I glanced around me, "Stephanie, what are you doing sitting here?" So I proceeded to stand up to get out of there, but I fell to the floor, realizing then my ability to walk was gone.

That day, being on my knees of that hospital floor, has been an extremely defining moment in my life. I made a promise to myself: I can and I will walk out of that hospital, no matter what I was being told. And I kept that promise to myself. The same faith, strength and determination that got me out of that coma state, walked me out of those hospital doors four months later on October 8, 1993.

Today that faith, strength and determination has been a bond to my life. Assisting me through many struggles from this brain injury, but also driving me to be as strong as possible. They have taken me as far as The Boston Marathon finish line.

Now 23 years after my accident, I give back by sharing the strength I cultivated from those hard moments, through a non-profit brain trauma organization I developed: Share Your Strong. I speak with children and individuals worldwide, providing encouragement to stay their course and keep faith so strong you can stand on it. I do this all through my testimony of the power of never giving up in life. I know for certain we are capable of moving mountains, because I have moved quite a few, and I am far from done yet.

Stephanie M. Freeman is a mother, a runner, but most importantly, a survivor, saying: Never Give Up, Never Give In, Never Stop Trying, Never EVER Give Up! *www.shareyourstrong.org*

Chapter Eighty
Post-Traumatic Stress Disorder and Traumatic Brain Injury – USMC

Stevena Pen
Saint Paul, Minnesota

2010 was a great year for me. After being honorably discharged from the Marine Corps in 2009, I lived in Palm Springs, California for a year. At the end of May 2010, I decided to move back to Minnesota to be closer to my family.

The Marine Corps changed my life through all the different experiences and traumatic events as part of the 2nd Battalion 7th Marines during 2006–2009. My first deployment was in Fallujah, Iraq, and my second deployment was to the Helmand province in Afghanistan.

After returning to my home state of Minnesota in 2010, my life was once again changed forever.

When I woke up in a hospital bed, I thought it was all a dream. Having been in a coma for months, I felt very lost when I woke up and heard beeps from machines and found tubes attached to me.

A cracked skull, frontal left and right side of my brain were all damaged. I had to learn how to walk, talk, and breathe all on my own again.

After months of rehab, I worked tirelessly as my goal to get back to "normal." I found out that I had a PTSD flashback and that led me to jump out of a moving car traveling over 30 miles per hour, twice.

Therapy visits went from three months as a daily inpatient, then to five days a week for about six months, then three days a week for about two years. After that, it was twice a week for about a year, then once a week for about six months.

Am I doing okay? No, not really, but I am doing a lot better than I was in 2010.

I now own a restaurant where I do all the public relation, media, and marketing. I have a handful of friends who I can trust. They and my family helped me get through my bad days.

Things are tough, life is hard, but if you are also living with post-traumatic stress disorder (PTSD) and a traumatic brain injury as a secondary injury, I think it's a miracle I'm still here. What I do know from all the love and support is that the people I associate with *do care*. They are the reasons why I'm here.

I want to thank the doctors, nurses, and specialist at the Hennepin County Medical Center, Veterans Affairs Medical Center, and Courage Kenny Rehabilitation Institute for helping put me back together.

Stevena was born in Minneapolis and raised in Saint Paul. While in the Marine Corps after high school, he has seen and done things no one could imagine. Follow, subscribe, and see some of the things he does and his journey though his recovery and success.
YouTube: Penaloo
Facebook: Kolap Restaurant
Website: www.KolapRestaurant.com

Chapter Eighty-One
Medical Resident Finds a New Life After Suffering Terrible Stroke

Summer Blackhurst
Kaysville, Utah

Will Blackhurst went to bed one night in 2008 after one of his long days of work in his first year of medical residency. To our knowledge he only complained of a headache once to a friend. It was early the next morning his alarm rang to wake him for his morning shift, but he did not respond to the call of the alarm. Will's roommate shut off the alarm so he could sleep, and then later left for work. Will remained unconscious in his bed. Co-workers knew something was wrong when Will didn't answer his phone. They drove to his apartment to find his car there, but no one answered the door. By the time they finally got his roommate to come unlock the door, Will had been unconscious for more than thirteen hours.

It took the doctors another day to figure out that Will had been hit with a hypothalamic stroke, and both sides of his brain had been affected. Will woke up a day after that. Words and walking did not come for another couple days. He was given a feeding tube until he was ready to start eating on his own. Will's mother and father and several siblings took turns flying into Columbus, Ohio, to stay with Will in the hospital.

When the stroke hit, Will was thirty years old, and doctors never were able to discover what caused the stroke or even where the clot came from. After more than a month in the hospital, Will flew home for outpatient treatment in Utah. It was here they repaired his Patent Foramen Ovael, a common heart condition, which is generally considered to be harmless.

I was the ex-girlfriend at the time. When I heard the news, I was driving and had to pull over to pray and wipe some tears. I couldn't believe it. After all that work in medical school and residency and all that school debt, he was thrown into a very difficult situation.

Initially Will slept. His memory of the year earlier was completely wiped away. His short-term memory was shot. His executive functioning and processing speed was severely hampered. Of course, sadness set in. Depression and denial were a piece of what he had to deal with up front, but it wasn't as difficult for him as it was for his parents and for me. He knew he wasn't a doctor, but he didn't realize that he wasn't going to get his job back. His parents and I were his caregivers, and we were a little more aware of the possible ramifications of his new conditions than he was at first.

We hoped that he would get back to his place in the residency rotation, but it was just really bad timing. He still needed to take another set of boards to finish his MD certification, and after the first year of healing, he could barely even write, let alone remember names or diseases or common aliments.

During his recovery, a lot of painful realities unraveled, the loss of a job, having to move back home, and so on. Of course there was incredible physical healing as the years passed, but even more phenomenal was a healing of the heart. The reasons that had kept us from being together before the stroke were gone. We now lived in the same state, and Will's commitment fears disappeared. My broken heart healed and sealed with his as we began to piece together his life, and I rediscovered my one true love.

Our love story is one for another day, but to be short, I can tell you, when love is real, it never dies, it is long suffering, it grows and grows, despite various trials and tribulations. With a little faith and trust, it can be better than before. Nine months after the stroke, Will and I were married. His healing journey was far from over. It took another six years for him to get a job working in health information at a hospital.

We have been married for almost eight years, and every year I can see healing. His abilities improve. He has no memory issues. He and I rarely battle over calendaring and planning like we did in the first few years. He has a small slur in his voice every now and then, but not near what it had been the first few years.

Together we have had three children who are our world. Will is the best dad. They have no idea what their father has been through. But the life that flows through their little beings is testament to the hope that can come after stroke.

The greatest challenges of possibly losing Will, and then waiting and waiting and waiting for his abilities to return, are a faint memory. His career is definitely different, but I know through experience now that *money does not happiness buy*. This family we have does. We recently bought a beautiful, but humble home with an amazing yard on the outskirts of Salt Lake City, Utah. Our healing came through faith—faith in our Heavenly Father and in one another. When fear could have paralyzed us both, it didn't because we believed God was watching over us, and He knew more than we did. Peace radiated from this difficult time, instead of tears and doubts.

Any time I spend with another survivor and or caregiver of stroke and TBI my heart hurts for them. Especially when they are in the thick of the recovery. I wish I could tell them to be still. Stay calm. Truth and light and healing will come. For Will, it took more years than we would have liked, but God knew what He was doing. Just know with faith, you'll be okay. God is great. He loves His children and will never leave them alone."

Summer Blackhurst married her on-again-off-again boyfriend of six years, a year after his stroke. Those first few years of marriage there was a lot of transition, but nothing prepared her for what she learned. Love conquers all; it heals. It is patient, kind, long suffering and with a little faith, they've learned they can both do hard things! They have been married eight years, and have three beautiful children. Finally, after all they have been through, they are more in love than ever. Read their entire story at www.willsrecovery.blogspot.com or following our continuing journey at www.whathappensinstead.blogspot.com

Chapter Eighty-Two
The Way the Wind Blows

Susan Cason Blackburn
Lagrange, Georgia

August 27, 2010 is a day I don't remember, but one that I'll never forget. That day the wind blew obstacles into my path, and many thought that I would never overcome these obstacles. I was driving with three of my children to pick up my oldest from school. An afternoon thunderstorm caused a huge rotten tree limb to fall onto my car as I was driving.

I have no recollection of the accident, but my children, twins, age 3, and the other, 7, will never hear thunder again without pictures creeping into their minds of their mom bent over the car's console.

I was transferred to a hospital in a bigger town close by, and had surgery that afternoon to remove clots from my brain. I was unresponsive for about eight weeks, but MRIs showed there was still brain activity, so my family was never given options to remove life support. When I started responding with thumbs-up signs, I was transferred to the awesome Shepherd Center in Atlanta. I have very few memories of the four months I was there in both inpatient and outpatient rehabilitation, so anything I know from that time is from looking at pictures and family stories.

In those four months, I went from no verbal communication, not eating, etc., to performing all Activities of Daily Living (ADL) independently. I was still in a wheelchair when I left because of hemiparalysis, but with about six months of rehab in my hometown, I went from a walker to a cane to completely independent walking.

Doctors had no explanation for my rapid recovery, but I did: it was all a miracle from the awesome God that I serve. The wind caused the limb to fall on my car, but it didn't stop there. After being home for a few months, the wind was knocked out of me when my husband of thirteen years told me that he and one of my closest friends had become very dependent on each other throughout the ordeal, and they couldn't be around each other anymore because the feelings were getting too intense—and they wanted to save their marriages. Needless to say, within eighteen months of my accident, we were divorced, and so was she. They married each other three years after the accident.

To me, this was the hardest part of my battle—having to fight in a courtroom to prove that I was capable of caring for my children alone. I believe my strength was possible only because of God's help. Six years later, I can say that I am on the road to complete physical and emotional recovery. I have been able to purchase a new house, and my children are with me every other week.

I would not be where I am without my family and God. Never give up. The wind blows, but TBI survivors are stronger than the wind.

Susan is a 43-year-old brain injury survivor from LaGrange, Georgia. She has four children, twins age 9, a 13-year-old, and a 17-year-old who are her life. Both her faith in God and her parents play an important role in her life.

Chapter Eighty-Three
Fighting Through It All

Tammy A. Martin
Stratford, Ontario, Canada

I have a condition that causes me to fall, or nearly fall, between five and twenty times a day. My initial head injury occurred in February of 2013, due to one of these falls. I tried to blow it off as being no different than the countless other times I had "bonked my head," but I quickly noticed it was not the same. My doctor ordered complete bed rest. No screen time, reading, music, *nothing!*

Also, and most heartbreaking for me, I had to send my children away. My doctor had said that if I didn't send them away to ensure I could really rest, then she would have to admit me to hospital so that she could be sure I rested. So my children left, for over three months. I experienced so many emotions during my rest. Some could be attributed to having my children away from me for the first time ever, but the rest was solely due to the head injury. I would have fits of self-hate, and I would rage at myself. I began to frantically cut myself with steak knives, over and over again, all up and down my legs, making both deep cuts and some were barely scratches. I wasn't thinking. I did it so many different times that I really don't know how many days it lasted. Did I want to die? No. I don't know what was happening inside of me, but I know that at no point did I want to die. I had the best things to fight for: my children.

A very obvious result of my head injury was a severe stutter. The doctor couldn't understand why it was there. No one could, but there it was. My family and my closer friends were very patient with me, but I was so very frustrated. As a person who was always known for clear and precise speech, it was so challenging to try to communicate. Often I would choose to say nothing at all, rather than to try to be understood. Obviously a number of people got tired of trying to be around me, so my social circle became smaller. The stutter lasted about three-and-a-half months. Suddenly when I woke one day—

after a terrible night of migraines that nearly had me going to the hospital—the stutter was *gone*. If I have a day that simply asked too much out of me, I am more likely to stutter a little bit here and there. I always freeze when it happens because I'm terrified it is back to stay.

I had always felt that I was the plain person, one who could easily be overlooked. I feel like I have lost my only unique aspect: my mind. My mind, my large vocabulary, my knowledge on various topics, was all that I had to be "special," but now it is gone. It's still very bad on most days. When I am very lucky and have rested a lot, I feel tendrils of the old me trying to bust through, and I get a lot of my mind back. But most days, doing the slightest thing requiring focus, or dealing with stress, or crowds, or too many sounds or sights or smells, or just *too much* of anything, I have to fight for my words.

I explained it once to my husband as "I'm sifting through muddy water, trying to find the word I want. I keep grabbing words, thinking it's the right one, only to have to drop it back into the water and to keep up my search." Going to the grocery store, and being asked how are you, is a struggle. I smile and try to act "natural," but then can't find the words, "I'm good, and you?" My anxiety that someone might speak to me has me nervous to go out in public. I am terrified that I will blunder somehow.

Since this initial bad fall, I have had two other falls that resulted in being placed back on bed rest, and also caused the stutter to return. Luckily, I did not resume the cutting. It was only about eighteen months from the first fall to the last one. And this was a fall that resulted in bed rest from a head injury. I still hit my head all the time. I now use a walker when I am out and about, to help me to have something slightly softer to land on, or when it is an "almost" fall, then I have something with which to catch myself. I am basically over being embarrassed about the walker. I do notice the judging glances from strangers. The look up and down my body, and the expression of "What's wrong with her?" I also have a helmet, but am incredibly resistant to wearing it because it bothers me a lot. I do try to remember it when doing stairs though, as I've been lucky so far that my falls downstairs have not hurt me too badly.

My memory is terrible. I have even accidentally stopped medications because I thought that I was supposed to. For example, I stopped anxiety meds when I was given new pain meds because somehow I thought the new pain meds were to replace the anxiety ones. I am trying to figure out a way around that. Figuring out ways around other things is the name of the game these days. I keep a lot of notes. I rely on voice memos. I text myself. I make lists. I like to colour code things, because when I glance, the colour helps to keep things separate. I can see each thing as an individual issue. I am so much better at asking for help now, which was something I was really struggling with at the start.

Not everything is bad, though.

About a month into my initial bed rest, I broke the rules and went on the phone. I called into a weight loss support group that I had been on before everything happened. Through that, I met my (now) husband. He moved 1200 miles to join me here. We have been married for over two years. He met me in the "after," so he knows fully what's going on. He has been a real gift in the darkness. He helps me to see that I have more to offer than just my mind, as I had believed all my life. He shows me where I am strong, and supports me when I need it. He doesn't try to coddle me, or anything like that. He helps as I need it, even if it's to simply show his support. He encourages me to find ways that I can do things, and to go into stores even though I am nervous. But when he can see I am *done* for the day (or week or month), then he doesn't push.

Also, my babies have been absolutely amazing. The two that were still living at home when everything started are now 17 and 16, and my oldest is 21. My younger two had to take on so many different responsibilities, from shopping to cleaning to keeping an eye on Mom. I am sad that they lost some youthful fun that kids should have, but they sure did it beautifully. I couldn't be any prouder as a Mom. They matured a little quicker than they should have had to, but we are also now a lot closer than I think we would have been otherwise.

Am I glad that I got hurt? No way. Would I change anything that came from it? I really don't think so. I am happy where all of my relationships are right now. I am thankful because some things would not have happened in my life or in my children's lives without my injury. I guess I kind of see it as the silver lining in the horrible storm that blew into our lives. Maybe it is just the way that I have found to be at peace—most of the time.

Every day is a struggle in one way or another—*but I am alive!*

Tammy is a wife, a mother, and a grandmother. She enjoys, above all else, spending time with her family and her little Chihuahua Lucy. Tammy has survived her injuries through the combined forces of sheer determination and being surrounded by the most loving and supportive family anyone could ask for.

Chapter Eighty-Four
Walk, Bang, Knockout

Tania Topping
Manawatu, New Zealand

Hello, let me introduce myself. My name is Tania Topping, a 35-year-old female who lives in New Zealand. I am a mother to two wonderful children; a son born in 2008, and a daughter born in 2013.

I have been employed in the same job since January 2002, doing an administration case progression role for a government organisation. I have enjoyed the full-time job as it made me feel like I am helping people.

I used to lead a busy but organised life, dropping my children off to care in the mornings, working full time from 8 a.m. to 4:30 p.m. five days a week, and then picking the children up to sort tea (have evening meal) and do their bedtime routines.

My life hit a roadblock on the 16th April 2015, when I was in a pedestrian crossing lane because the green light told me to walk. The crossing was the only thing separating me from a straight 10-minute walk to my car. I ended up riding a woman's car bonnet/hood a couple of metres down the street.

Yes, I am very lucky in that I still have all my functions, but it is extremely frustrating not being allowed or able to do things that I remember I had been capable of doing. Fatigue is my biggest hurdle.

Unfortunately for me, the intersection cameras did not record me being hit by the car. The cameras only showed condensation (due to rain earlier that day)—and my bright blue handbag flying across the screen.

For me, it's all felt like it happened to someone else, and I'm the one who is having to deal with the consequence. Sometimes I feel like I'm arguing just to be able to make decisions for myself.

The police decided there was an issue with the intersection lights. The detective filmed herself crossing that same crossing three times, and she almost got hit by a car. Apparently the green man indicating "walk" went green at the same time as the green light telling the car to go, but vehicles forget to give way to those walking across the crossing.

Apparently there's not enough evidence to charge the driver with reckless driving, causing injury.

Me on the other hand...I've been sentenced to walking the footpath with my children in tow, having been stopped from driving until health professionals see fit to allow me to undertake a driving assessment.

I've been told the driver did not see me until I was on her window screen/windshield, which makes me wonder what the hell was she looking at if it wasn't out her window screen, which was shattered by my impact with it. I've been told (as if it's meant to reduce what she did to me) that the driver held my hand while waiting for emergency assistance to arrive.

I was flown by air ambulance to Wellington Hospital that night back in April when the car hit me. I ended up with a neck fracture and a severe traumatic brain injury. The neurosurgeons that night did emergency surgery on me, and took the front right-hand quarter of my skull away to enable the swelling of my brain to go down. My skull piece was placed in the freezer at Wellington Hospital.

I suffered 22 days of post-traumatic amnesia, during which I have been told I spent two weeks at Wellington Hospital, and then I was transferred to a rehab in Porirua.

When I first remembered waking up in rehab in the middle of May 2015, I did not freak out about where I was. I got out of the rehab bed and walked down a corridor, but was shocked when the nurses said hello and called me by name because I had no idea who they were. But I adjusted well to being in rehab, and accepted that I had to be there.

I was equipped with a lovely neck brace, which I had to wear all the time, and a black rugby helmet to wear during the day, to protect me from any random tackles from strangers.

Apparently when I first got to rehab, I fought verbally to remove the neck brace, but after waking up from my amnesia, I reluctantly accepted that I had to wear it. I wore the neck brace six weeks, before an x-ray showed that the neck fracture had healed. It was such a relief to throw it in the rubbish bin. I had to endure the rugby helmet for three months until I had surgery to have the removed part of my skull returned in July 2015.

The looks I got from strangers because I was wearing the black helmet were amazing. My confidence to talk to strangers grew, and I happily said hello if people looked at me. A security guard at the shopping centre in Porirua asked me, "How was training?" He thought I had been to rugby training. Anyone who knows me would just crack up laughing at this idea.

For five of my seven weeks in rehab, I shared a four-person hospital-like room with only one other woman. She was wonderful and saved me a seat in the dining room for each meal. She helped me adjust to being there.

For the last two weeks of my stay, I had a single room to myself, as I had progressed extremely well in my recovery and didn't need lots of attention from the nurses.

Overall rehab was nice because I was made to feel welcomed and included. I was given a weekly calendar with my various appointments. We had a lot of down time during the day, so during my time in rehab, I read three novels and gave the reception staff a helping hand between having naps. There wasn't much else to do, and I had lost interest in watching television.

It was really hard to deal with being three hours away from my family and friends. Facebook helped me reconnect with the world outside rehab.

I got lost a bit walking around in rehab, as the corridors all looked the same. I suggested to my occupational therapist that the walls should have signs so that patients wouldn't get lost. Shortly, she brought me blank paper and some felt-tips. Then I handwrote twelve signs I stuck to the walls. After a couple of weeks of these signs being up, I was allowed to use the computer, so I typed and laminated them. It was wonderful knowing I had left my mark at rehab.

To help me with being able to cook again, I was given $10 once a week and taken to the supermarket. I had to plan a meal to make just for me for lunch the following day, and buy what I needed to make it. The only rule was you had to use the oven to cook it. I found this exercise extremely hard, because cooking for just me is not easy, having cooked for my partner and children for years, and I never really cooked hot lunches before.

On the 15 July 2015, after being frozen for three months, my skull part was returned to me. Luckily this time it was only a short three-night stay in hospital, after a three-hour operation.

I was fortunate enough to be released to go straight home after my surgery, without having to go back to rehab. This was just in time for my son to return to my full-time care, and to start Term 3 at our local school. I had to change his school so I could make sure he got to school each day, and with me not being able to drive, it had to be within walking distance.

My confidence to do things has taken its toll, especially cooking. I have trouble determining what needs to be cooked first so it all can be dished together and still be hot. I love the slow cooker because it helps me out as I can just throw lots of things in at once and leave it for four hours.

My navigation abilities have gone out the window. I need to look at a map and ask strangers for directions if I can't figure out where I'm trying to go. It is slowly improving, but it will take time.

Accident Compensation Corporation (ACC) is the sole and compulsory provider of accident insurance in New Zealand for all work and non-work injuries. I am extremely thankful that this organisation exists. ACC are helping me out while I cannot work, including paying for me to travel to and from the city by taxi, along with funding my recovery team that includes my occupational therapist, social worker, psychologist, home care giver and the physiotherapist.

I believe that without these wonderful people, my recovery would have been a lot harder.

Being back at home has been both joyful and hard. Besides having myself to look after, I also had my children to care for. I have noticed that I cannot handle large levels of noise. I've recently completed the Incredible Years Parenting Course to up my skills.

In September 2015, I was allowed to go back to work after a five-month break. Work and ACC had established that I would go in to read the newsletter to be kept up to date with any changes, and to socialise with my co-workers for morning tea.

I miss being able to be productive, and miss the conversations I used to have with my co-workers about the files and actual work. Sometimes I've wondered what is the point of going in to read the newsletter because no one ever talks to me about it.

I underwent a neurological assessment on the 14 December 2015. The results came out in January 2016. The report writer is recommending that I *not* work or drive at this time. It was a really numb feeling getting the results, and it's just added to the things I have no control over since the accident.

In March 2016, I started volunteering two mornings a week at my son's school, to help me deal with my fatigue. I have really enjoyed this, and it has given me a great reason to leave the house. The teachers have been giving me reading books to file away, and work to be laminated.

After a year of reading the newsletter at work once a week, the company has now ended my employment with them. I feel really sad because it's a job that I loved doing, but due to the doctor's recommendations (that basically my recovery to go back to full-time employment is unknown), my employer cannot keep a job open for me anymore.

I feel like I survived for my children, and the reality now for me is to live every day as best as I can, and you can only do that, too. It's easier to do if you surround yourself with people who help you smile.

Tania used to work full-time and care for her two children, until a routine walk to her vehicle, and an unwanted car bonnet (hood) ride turned her life upside down. While recovering from her severe traumatic brain injury, Tania's stubbornness has enabled her to take her new life and challenges as they are, to enable her to succeed so far in being able to watch her children grow and enjoy the small things that she missed out on before. It's not her intelligence or decision making that's gone, just that getting the results take more attempts and effort than ever before, but with that Tania has risen to the challenge, with a strength and determination she had previously hidden deep down.

Chapter Eighty-Five
My TBI: Moment-by-Moment

Ted Morin
New York City, New York

I live in New York City and teach movement to actors at a professional acting conservatory. I had a near-fatal motorcycle accident in November of 2011, resulting in multiple physical injuries and my TBI.

It was early spring when I was discharged from the hospital, almost four months after my accident.

It wasn't until I got home that I began to understand not only had I been in a coma for a month, broken my leg and fractured my spine in multiple places, but I had also broken my brain. Nothing felt real to me. Everything I did felt both familiar and strange, like I was doing it for the first time in my life.

I walked on a *tightrope of uncertainty* every day, all day. The only thing that felt real to me, that I was certain of, was the present moment. Staying present and in the moment gave me a sense of stability. Everything else was a blurry, scrambled mess. The inside of my head was like a library turned upside down, books scattered everywhere, stacked on top of each other, some open, some closed, books turned this way and that, torn pages, stacks and stacks of books. There's a lot of information, but it's a jumbled mess. I held onto each moment like a buoy you would grasp onto were you lost at sea.

In the hospital I had constant care, but when I came home all that came to an abrupt end. When I was released from the hospital I had to learn how to live on my own. I don't remember how I got up the single flight of sixteen steps to the door of my apartment on the first floor of my brownstone. I'm sure my best friend, Walter, was behind me, should I fall back, and my friend Alex was beside me, his arm hooked in mine. I was unable to walk down the steps for several weeks. I had to sit at the top of the stairs and slide down on my butt if I wanted to go outside for a walk.

A home-care nurse came three times a week to do physical therapy with me on my bed, in my apartment, and down the hallway of the first floor of my building. I had a lot of time on my hands, not working, and not being able to manage much around the house. My balance was bad. I couldn't lift things or bend over to pick something up should I drop it. I had to move slowly so as not to fall.

Because I lived alone, as time went on, I had to do everything myself. I had to dress myself, buy my own groceries, make my meals and feed myself, shower and clean up, pay the rent and my bills, plus I had to do the exercises the therapists in outpatient treatment told me to do. Alex would often stay with me for few days, clean my apartment, make my dinners, and always made sure I was comfortable.

Not only did I have to do everything myself, I had to figure out *how to do it*. My brain would get exhausted after doing the simplest of tasks. Taking a shower was physical work, having to balance, bend and reach, and my brain would get worn out before my body. I had to constantly think of what to do next, decide what product to use and on what part of my body, how to comb my hair, floss my teeth and trim my beard. By the time I was done, I'd have to lie down and take a nap. Surrendering the weight of my head to the pillow was a huge relief. My brain felt like Jell-O settling back and down into the mold of my skull. The earth had never felt as good, as comforting. Gravity had never felt so important.

I knew I had to go back to work. My financial situation wouldn't have it any other way, and I had no one to take care of me. Having to go to work got me out of bed in the morning, walking and moving and living for myself again. There were no more doctors, nurses and therapist of every flavor cheering me on, rooting for me. I was the only one who could do the work, who could summon up the courage and the strength to try, or not. The choice was entirely my own.

The doctors would often comment that it was a good thing I knew so much about the body, how it moves and functions. I'm sure it helped when I was learning how to sit, stand, and walk. Ironically though, it's not all that knowledge of the body that got me through each day—it was the first exercise I teach my students when they start to study with me, the first exercise they do in every class I teach. It's this exercise that gets me out of bed in the morning, out the door to walk my dog, eat breakfast, shower, dress, and commute to work. It's what enables me to navigate my way though New York City.

At the start of class, I have my students lie on the floor on their back and allow their bodies to come to a lengthened, simple, neutral place. I ask them to uncross their arms, uncross their legs, their hair, fingers, eyes and teeth. "Surrender the weight of your entire body to the surface of the floor," my voice is soft; the lights in the studio are dimmed. "Allow gravity to do what gravity does very well…it holds you up. Trust the earth, the planet. You do not have to anything about your breath. You especially don't have to take a breath. There's enough air in the room for all of us, and your body knows exactly how to breathe, when to breathe, so you don't have to think about that."

Once the class is set up, I start the exercise.

"There's nothing you need to do during the next few minutes of time. Can you simply be present with your body and the way it feels right here, right now, in this moment? Simply notice the experiences that are alive in your body. Can you free yourself from judging whatever you notice; from having to fix anything, adjust anything, alter anything? You don't have to feel better or worse. Simply accept the experiences that you notice, good, bad or otherwise."

I stop talking and give them a few minutes to participate in the process.

Many students get fidgety; they twitch and scratch and adjust themselves. Some curl over onto their side to get more comfortable. Some of them drift off, start thinking, fantasizing, daydreaming; some of them even fall asleep. When I start speaking again, the sound of my voice serves as a reminder that they are in class, participating in an exercise that's both simple and challenging. I tell them this is the most important exercise they will learn in the two years of movement classes they will have with me.

"You can always begin from wherever you are, but you need a moment to become aware of where you are, how you're feeling, and what's going on. When you can accept that, you're in the perfect place to begin your work as an actor, an artist."

I might pause and give them a moment to connect with the concept, before continuing.

"This exercise is a both a gift and a curse. It's a gift to know that you can always begin from wherever you are, and it's a curse because there are no excuses."

My brain never feels like it's in the right place to begin. I never feel like I want to or that I can. I have to remind myself that I don't have to feel any particular way in order to start my day, in order to do the next task that's in front of me: get out of bed, walk my dog, feed Buster breakfast, feed myself, shower, dress, plan my classes, leave the apartment, walk to the subway and ride it to midtown, walk through Time Square to get to the studio, organize myself and my notes, walk into my class, open my mouth and speak the first words. It all feels completely impossible and overwhelming to me.

I have to remind myself that it's all right for me to feel the way I'm feeling.

I have to remind myself that I am always in the perfect place from which to begin.

My actual return to work was a slow process. After a few months, I felt confident commuting to the studio on my own. I had practiced going up and down stairs with my cane so I could manage commuting on the subway. For the first few weeks I would go and observe one of my colleagues teaching an acting class, and then I'd observe my assistant who was now teaching all the movement classes on the schedule since my accident. I started to reconnect with what it was that I did for a living. Going to work was like going on an adventure, the way going to physical therapy sessions felt when I was in the hospital, re-entering the world from a coma. I never knew what to expect, and was always thrilled when I could do something with my body that I wasn't able to do the previous session.

At work, I started to teach short exercises in some of the movement classes. At first, I could only teach for a few minutes before my thoughts would drift off and away from what I was doing. My brain would get exhausted from the exertion of having to concentrate on what I was saying, and on what to say next. I asked the studio to buy me a stool on wheels that I could use to move around the class. It was easier and less cumbersome to teach sitting down than standing and walking with a cane. Often, students were doing physical exercises on the floor. I wasn't able to bend over without falling, but when sitting, their bodies were closer so I could use my hands to make adjustments or corrections.

I gradually increased my stamina to stay focused, and was able to get through an entire class. My assistant was there to fill in should I need to take a break or lie down or take a nap because my brain was exhausted. And then, one day, I told him not to come to class. I knew I had to be able to do it on my own if I was going to survive in New York City. I had to work—and my work was teaching.

One night, when I got home from the studio, Alex came over. We were having dinner and watching the Westminster Dog Show. I love dogs. The Cairn Terrier was being judged. The handler brought the dog up to the judge's table, who then did his usual inspection. The dog was put down on the ground and the handler walked the dog on the runway while the judge watched, nodding his head, his face expressionless. The announcer; however, was lively as ever: "The Cairn Terrier. A little dog with a big-dog attitude," he said, and then he concluded the segment with: "No man would ever be embarrassed being seen walking a Cairn." These two comments got etched in my scrambled, messed-up brain.

One of my doctors had suggested I get a dog, saying, "A dog would be really good therapy for you. You should think about it."

I hadn't thought about getting a dog until I saw the Cairn Terrier and heard the announcer's comments, but then I became obsessed. I started to look for breeders who had puppies for sale or were expecting litters. In late June, Wally drove me to a breeder in Connecticut who had a litter of five, three females and two males. The three females and one of the males were already sold, but the buyers of the male hadn't chosen which pup they were taking. If I got there before them, I would have first choice.

When we arrived, the breeder let all the dogs out in the back yard. I made my way to a chair, set my cane down and watched them play. The puppies were scrambling around as puppies do, jumping here, leaping there, snarling, barking and carrying on. It was a hot and humid day. There was a big metal bowl filled with water in the yard. I looked over and saw a tiny pup sitting right in the middle of the bowl. He looked like he was smiling, as if to say: "Run you idiots, run all you like. I'm going to sit right here where it's cool."

A warm, familiar feeling came over me as I remembered the day I met a dog when I was in intensive care.

I was lying in my hospital bed, my room empty, no visitors, no nurses, and no doctors poking and prodding their way around my busted-up body. I closed my eyes and could feel myself sink into the mattress that continually adjusted to my body by inflating and deflating in various locations. Apparently, it was some high-tech hospital bed meant to decrease the risk of bedsores. Every time I would adjust my position, the mattress would conform to take the pressure off those points in my body that were bearing my weight. It was like the mattress and my body were having a conversation.

I heard someone enter the room, a shuffling of feet and a clicking sound, like toenails coming into contact with the floor. I opened my eyes and saw an older woman standing close to my bed holding a leash. My eyes followed the leash from her hand down toward the floor, and to my surprise, a dog was sitting there. He looked like he was smiling, like he belonged in a cartoon.

"Hi," the woman said. "My name is June, and this is Dante. Dante is a therapy dog, and we thought we'd stop by to see how you were doing today."

"Therapy dog?" I had never heard of a therapy dog.

"Yes," she replied. "Dante is trained to be of comfort to those who both need it and are open to dogs. Do you like dogs?"

"I love dogs."

"Would you like to meet Dante?"

"Sure!" Dante's smile brightened when I agreed, as if he understood what we're talking about.

June picked Dante up and gently placed him at the foot of my hospital bed. He looked at me, as if to ask permission, and then walked towards me and lay down, his little body snuggling into my side, his head resting on my lap. He never took his eyes off me. He was so calm, so present, so affectionate. I placed my hand on his head and began to gently slide it down the nape of his neck and along his spine. I was fascinated by the touch of his fur, his shape, and his smile. Dante intuitively knew that he could trust me.

"What kind of dog is he?"

"He's a King Charles Spaniel."

I gave Dante my full attention. It felt good to touch his soft coat, to feel his little body breathe, to feel his heart beating underneath my palm.

"Hey Dante, wanna come up? Come."

Dante slowly and gently crawled onto my chest and laid down again, his little head resting on my shoulder. Now I could stroke the full length of his body, from the top of his head all the way down to his tail. He closed his eyes, and I closed mine, while I continued to pet my newfound friend.

"Well look at you two. A match made in heaven." June chuckled at the cleverness of her comment.

I didn't respond. Dante began to snore.

Now months later, this little Cairn puppy sitting in the water dish was smiling just like Dante. I pointed to the pup and asked the breeder if he was available. I knew he was the dog for me. As luck would have it, he was one of the two males I could pick from. I returned the following week, and Buster has been with me ever since.

The doctor was right. Buster became a focal point for me. I had to organize his day, his walks, his meals, his playtime, his naps, and housebreaking. He became the most important thing in my life. He filled my time, and in retrospect that was the best therapy for me as I started to reconnect with life. I had no time to think about myself. Unstructured time was my worst enemy, and in many ways still is. Buster not only gave my days structure, he was with me when I learned how to walk without a cane. Sometimes, when lying in bed he would jump up and lay down on my chest, even snuggle his head into the crevice of my neck. In those moments, I always remember meeting Dante in the hospital that day.

Ted Morin is a Certified Movement Analyst who lives in New York City and teaches movement to actors at a professional acting conservatory. He was in a near-fatal motorcycle accident in 2011 resulting in his TBI and multiple physical injuries. He is currently writing a novel and hopes to give readers the opportunity to look through the eyes of someone living with a TBI.

Chapter Eighty-Six
Ten Things I Learned to Help Someone With a TBI

Toni Popkin
Alexandria, Virginia

Before my first TBI, I worked full time, first for about 25+ years as a licensed optician in Virginia; then at age fifty, I went back to school and received a certification in Mental Health as a Peer Support Provider. I worked in this field until my first TBI.

I sustained my fourth concussion less than a month ago during the summer of 2016. Unlike the other that involved someone crashing into my car, this was in my home. I passed out in the bathroom, hitting my head. It's a totally different type of injury with totally different symptoms, yet the recovery for all was basically the same. This last was a direct hit to the front of my head, whereas in the car crashes, my whole brain got bounced around.

My first TBI was in 2005 when a car full of teens crashed into the passenger side of my car. Then a lot was not yet known about concussions and TBIs. I frequently heard, "Be thankful you aren't as badly hurt as the passenger in your car who had already had a previous TBI." There was the common belief that you were really either bad off or okay, but nothing in between. I "looked" okay to most casual observers. Therefore I was left to my own devices to deal with my symptoms. No one suggested treatment because I wasn't "really bad."

However my life slowly fell apart. In 2008, almost three years post-accident, when I was hospitalized for a totally unrelated problem, a doctor started putting 2+2 together—and referred me for an evaluation by Brain Injury Services in Northern Virginia. Almost immediately I started receiving services to start putting my life back together. I learned compensatory skills, met others like myself who looked okay, and received in-home support for the hidden disaster no one knew was there.

Only I knew. I knew how I used to be, and how different I was now. I also knew most of my old friends had left me because they did not believe me when I would say I was having problems and needed help. I can't tell you how many times I'd be told, "I just saw you doing X; if you can do that, you surely don't need help with Y." What they didn't see was that I put so much effort into doing X that I had no reserve in my energy bank to take care of almost everything else.

Slowly, very slowly over the next several years I made a lot of progress in many areas. I began volunteering, teaching crafts to others with disabilities, which I loved. I became a very involved member of Brain Injury Services Speakers Bureau, and could tell I was making an impact when a person who I didn't recognize saw me in my sweats in a local pizza place—and commented on what I had said *a year before*! I was sharing my story of what it's like to live with a TBI in order to educate and to advocate.

In 2012, I was in another crash, this one more serious. A woman was making an illegal lane change, didn't see my car and crashed into it. She even told the police officer she was sorry that she didn't see me. Only much, much later did I learn she was not cited nor was a report written because the police had not witnessed it! Many of the gains I had made were lost. So was my faith in the justice system and in insurance companies, but that's for another story.

When people hear of someone having a TBI, I hear two main responses: "I wish I lived closer so I could do something," or "Call me if you need anything."

I will be the first, but probably not only one, to tell you open-ended questions are hard—they are hard for someone with a TBI at any stage, but especially when it is recent. A quote from a good friend of mine, artist Joanne Fink, on her blog, From Grief to Gratitude: "Provide practical assistance. Don't say 'call me if you need anything'... people who are sick/grieving are often disoriented and have trouble remembering things. They may not even remember that you offered to help, and even if they do remember, they probably won't want to impose on you."

"Rest" means you need to rest both your body and mind. It means very limited use of electronic devices, TV, or loud noise. Doing things for myself is hard right now. Many people like me live alone, and we need help from others.

Here is how you can help someone rest and recover, even when he seems okay. Here are my 10 practical ideas for helping a friend or loved one who has had a recent TBI.

- Call and say, "I'm on my way to the grocery store and am bringing you bread, eggs and milk. What else do you need?"
- Same for "I'm going to (wherever restaurant) and bringing you dinner, is there anything special you'd like or don't like"?
- Order carryout to be delivered even if you can't personally make or take something. This can be done even long distance. Almost every city has many restaurants that deliver other food, in addition to pizza and Chinese. Google "restaurant delivery" in that city.
- Do you have medicine that needs to be picked up? Where do you get it? I'm going to be at (fill in the place), so can I get it for you?
- Do you have any upcoming doctor appointments I can drive you to?
- May I come help you walk the dog, or pick up dog or cat food for you? What times do you walk your dog?
- What type book or magazine do you like? And then bring it or send it.
- I'd like to come visit for a few minutes, is tomorrow afternoon a good time? Be specific. While there, ask, "Is it okay that I water your plants, take out your trash, etc.?
- You probably haven't felt up to doing laundry or cleaning. May I come this weekend to do it for you?
- Call to just say, "Hi, I wanted to see how you are feeling." Make it brief if she says she is tired. Ask if calling or emails are better, and respect her request. Also ask is there a better time to call, like not before _____ a.m. or after _____ p.m.

Right after this last concussion, I received offers for help and food, and had visitors almost every day. Then after ten days, it stopped. I'm only guessing it stopped because someone who came to visit told others that "she looks good." I'll probably never know. What I do know is the help I desperately needed dried up too soon.

I truly wish people could find a small place in their busy lives to be empathetic to the needs of someone they know, not jumping to a conclusion just because I was able to take a shower that day. I wish they would consider the fact that I live alone, and have no family, spouse, or significant other near me to count on when I need something.

This latest concussion is so fresh that my emotions are very raw; this in itself causes more problems of feelings of loneliness and rejection. As my neurologist told me, "You've been down this road before, you probably know it better than I do." This is actually a very wise statement. Unless you've been down this road and experienced it, one can never fully appreciate how difficult it can be.

However, his message was something else—one of hope! Yes, this is my fourth time down this road. I've learned a lot. I've offered others a great gift in sharing what I've learned. I've advocated, educated, and raised my voice for those who are unable to. Each time my hope is that I touch just one person like I did with the person in the pizza shop.

Right now as I am feeling really sick, it's hard to remember this. I think I'll make myself a reminder note: ***"Remember how far I have come!"***

Toni Popkin lives with her full-service dog, Bud, in Northern Virginia. She has had three Traumatic Brain Injuries (TBIs) as results of auto crashes, none her fault, and a very recent concussion from passing out and hitting her head. She is an avid advocate for people with invisible disabilities like herself, educating and raising awareness by being a part of the Speakers Bureau for Brain Injury Services (www.braininjurysvcs.org) in Northern Virginia for the past six years. In her spare time, Toni loves making BUD Vases, doing crafts, and teaching others the joy of creativity. BUD Vases are the name of the handcrafted artisan vases she makes. They are decoupage glass vases made with handmade Thai paper and can hold fresh flowers or are used as décor.

Chapter Eighty-Seven
Finding My New Normal

Wendy Squire
Prince George, British Columbia, Canada

I was pumped when I skated onto the ice Halloween night, 2010; the women's hockey league season had just started, and I was more than ready for a good year. Following a divorce and some serious health issues, I was finally feeling good. Even my career as an RN was on track, and I was making plans for my future.

I was not expecting to find myself sliding on my back, headfirst down the ice. We hadn't even finished the first period. It felt like I hit a brick wall; my chest ached; my jaw wouldn't open; and I wondered if I'd broken my back. Apparently an opposing player, literally half my age and half my size, ran into me and shoved me. I'm told my feet left the ice as I flew backwards, and my head bounced when it hit the ice. I wanted to stand right up but my teammates slowed me down. Good thing, because I was very wobbly, and still couldn't figure out what was happening. The spectators and players all cheered and banged their sticks as I was assisted to the bench. Weird.

No one said I shouldn't, so I finished the game, taking long breaks between shifts. My head hurt, and I didn't feel right, but I had no idea how injured I was. I had yet to learn that with a concussion, *you are not able to assess yourself.* I just kept doing all the things I was responsible for doing, like going to work because I didn't get paid when I wasn't working.

A CT scan showed I didn't have a bleed, but I was told I had a concussion, and to take a few days off. Then I was told I had a serious concussion, and to take a few weeks off. Then it was post-concussion syndrome, which would take several months to heal. My expectation was always that I would get better. Completely.

Concentrating was a challenge, and my headaches worsened throughout the day. My skull felt several sizes too small for my brain. It felt very heavy, and at the same time like it was floating. I was in a fog. I felt off, not quite right. My dreams were vivid, and most nights I woke up gasping from nightmares. I napped daily for 90 minutes and longer. Evidently I looked fine, but I felt very, very different.

Few friends were able to be honest and open with me. Years later I realized that my friends and family suffered, too, watching me change and struggle. The brain injury affected more than just me. A nurse friend told me I had become melancholy and slow with my responses that used to be whip-fast. She noticed me touching things to check and maintain my balance, saying I acted stoned. It was actually reassuring to hear this. Despite being frightening, it was validating.

I was working very hard to do daily-living activities. The number and variety of symptoms was, and still is, amazing and sobering. Sometimes just brushing my teeth before bed felt deserving of Olympic gold.

After six months, I was able to work a full workload three days a week, with recovery days in between. Even though I usually needed acetaminophen to make it through, I'd definitely improved. My doctor decided I could try working full time in May, eight months after my fall.

Driving down my alley only a few weeks before I was to try full-time work, a neighbour backed out of his driveway and into my driver's door. I felt like a bobble-head doll with no control on where my head was bouncing. Getting out of the car, I went around to the back, relieved to see no damage to my rear bumper. It wasn't as bad as I thought! Stepping to the side, I noticed my very dented door. I swore softly and slowly. It wasn't about my car; it was about the damage to my brain. I knew I wasn't thinking properly. Everything was surreal, and I didn't know what to do.

April 11, 2011 was a life-changing date. The first injury interrupted my life, but this second one, I would discover, changed it.

Two years, the specialists said, was how long it took for a brain to heal. After that, there would be little significant improvement. I put my plans on hold, worked hard to heal—and then, after two years, I would carry on with my life. I could do this. I would be fine. My life plans would need a minor adjustment, but that's all. I would find ways to work around the challenges.

I wore purple-tinted glasses to help with my light sensitivity, and earplugs or filters for the sound issues. I made lists and used fridge magnets to remember things. My former "normal" of reading up to five books at a time dropped to one graphic novel at a time. I still met with my writers' group; seeing these friends was my one sure thing every two weeks, and I hung on to it. However, being part of or on the edge of multiple-person conversations was exhausting and induced headaches.

I had lost the ability to picture images in my mind, and words were no longer readily available so I couldn't imagine what I was writing. My physiotherapist suggested randomly posing my wooden drawing model, studying it for 30 seconds; then without looking at it, draw it. Easy enough I thought, but when I put pencil to paper, I had nothing. I couldn't remember, let alone picture where the arm or anything else was. This was horrifying. This was akin to losing an appendage. I didn't cry or yell because *emotionally I was flat*.

My biggest challenge was lack of energy and little stamina. I was irritable and touchy, but my friends were gracious—and I was oblivious. Just because they don't understand, doesn't mean they don't care and aren't hurting, too. It was years before I learned that they suffered losses in this too, plus they had to deal with me

Then I discovered woodcarving, something I'd wanted to try since I was a little girl. Carving was like I've taken my brain to the spa. I carved for hours each day. My writers' group came and did an intervention in my little patio, making it green and beautiful for me. My ability to concentrate and focus improved, and eventually I began to imagine things again.

Invisible injuries are hard. I just wanted to be understood—wanted someone to realize how much effort it took to do the simplest things. My boss said, "It must be nice to have all that time off." I eventually learned it isn't other people's responsibility to understand or care. I can choose to lose my expectations, rather than get angry or bitter.

At the two-year mark, I was still not doing well. I felt I'd plateaued in my recovery. Working two days a week was reduced to one day. I really loved where I worked, and who I worked with, but my career was slipping away. My funds were rapidly disappearing.

On my 50th birthday, I packed my things, and what was left of my life, into boxes. When people wondered why I would leave my beautiful, sunny home to live in the north with its long, cold winters, I would say that my mom lived there. They assumed I would be taking care of her. I didn't bother to correct them. Worst birthday ever.

It was a good move. I found a brain injury support group where I learned what really happened, and what can be done to work around it. It was helpful beyond words to meet other TBI survivors, to be understood and validated. It was empowering to see others improving, as well as people I could encourage.

Mom took care of grocery shopping, cooking and even the cleaning. I took care of me and attended support and teaching sessions. I rested and exercised, and gradually moved off my plateau.

Five years later I've accepted that I'll never be a nurse again. I've gone from a ten-minute shuffle around the block to a thirty-minute hard climb up steep hills, and from reading Peanuts to adult novels, though not Tolkien. I've developed systems and habits to make my life easier to handle. I've learned to look forward to the things I can do, rather than backwards at what I lost.

Two years means nothing. Recovery from a brain injury is frustratingly slow and discouragingly non-linear, but there is a new normal—and it is worth the effort to find. I've learned invaluable lessons that I wouldn't trade. People and my relationships with them are the most important things. Energy is still a precious commodity.

My new normal has good days, which I enjoy and value, and bad days, which I know will pass. I am a survivor!

Wendy Squire was a registered nurse before her TBIs, and writing was one of her favourite hobbies. She has continued to pursue this despite the new challenges, and is pleased to be published in several anthologies. She now lives with her mom and two cats in northern British Columbia, Canada.

Resources

Here is a small list of resources that I have compiled. These are sites that I have found helpful in my recovery, plus the one I created. I hope that they steer you in the right direction.

Brain Injury Association of America
www.biausa.org

Brain Injury Alliance (each state has one, I am listing the Minnesota site)
www.braininjurymn.org

Brain Line
www.brainline.org

Faces of TBI Podcast Series
www.blogtalkradio.com/facesoftbi
also available on iTunes

Facebook — The TBI Tribe
www.facebook.com/groups/792052120888627

Faces of TBI
www.facesoftbi.com

TBI Hope & Inspiration (sign up for their free digital magazine)
www.tbihopeandinspiration.com

International Resources

Canada Brain Injury Association
www.biac-aclc.ca/
10 Provincial Associations listed on their website

Australian Brain Injury Groups
www.braininjuryaustralia.org.au/
www.braininjury.org.au/portal/index.php

England – Headway
www.headway.org.uk/home.aspx

Headway – Ireland
www.headway.ie/

Ireland – Brain Injury Advocacy and Support
www.briireland.ie/bri/Main/Home.htm

Head Injury Society of New Zealand
www.head-injury.org.nz/

International Brain Injury Association
www.internationalbrain.org

European Brain Injury Society – this is more of an organization for professionals
www.ebissociety.org/

European Federation of Association of Families
www.bif-ec.eu/

European Brain Injury Consortium
www.ebic.nl/welcome.htm

Latin American Brain Injury Consortium
www.labic.org/

Meet the Cover Models

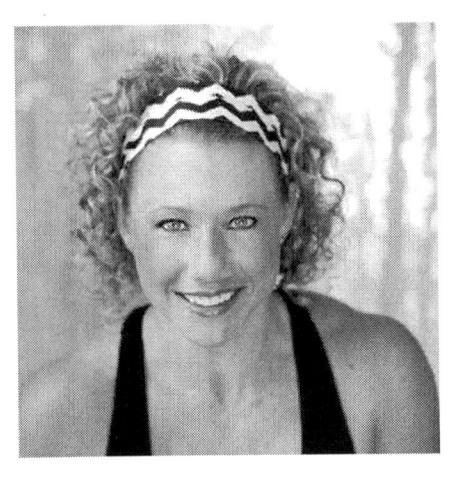

Belinda Clary
Belinda, from St. Paul, Minnesota, is a very active wife and mother of eight, small business owner, group fitness instructor, personal trainer, swim coach, deacon in her church, and competitive power lifter. She was affected by a TBI/concussion after a car accident in 2012. The road to "finding her new normal" has been long and challenging, but hasn't stopped her from striving for both personal and business successes and happiness in life. Belinda has such a love for life and the people around her that some say it is as infectious as her smile.

Heather L. George
Heather lives in St. Paul, Minnesota, and has been recognized for her work in adult education and instructional technology. Following her 2012 and 2014 brain injuries, she has focused on assistive technology and PCS awareness, research, and rehabilitation.

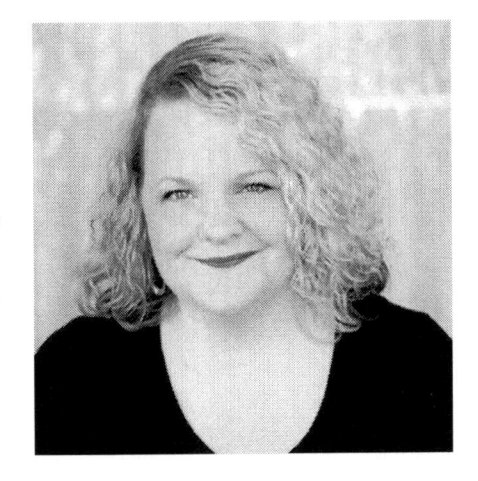

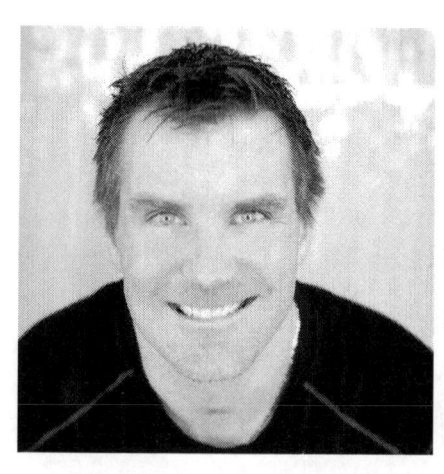

Nick Dennen

Nick is an inspiring author, speaker, and, first and foremost, a husband and father of two—who would not be here had he not been injured. He has a strong purpose of serving the greater good. His mission is to recognize the value of personal relationships while focusing on a positive attitude and heightening the awareness of traumatic brain injury. His motto is simple: anything really is possible if you believe. Anything!

Nikki Abramson

Nikki is the author of the books "I Choose Hope" in 2014 and "Hope for Today" in 2016, as well as co-author for a one hour one-woman play, "No Limits." She is a teacher, actor, speaker, and mentor who strives to bring hope and positivity to the world specifically in the areas of disabilities and adoption. Check out www.NikkiAbramson.com for more information on her story and work.

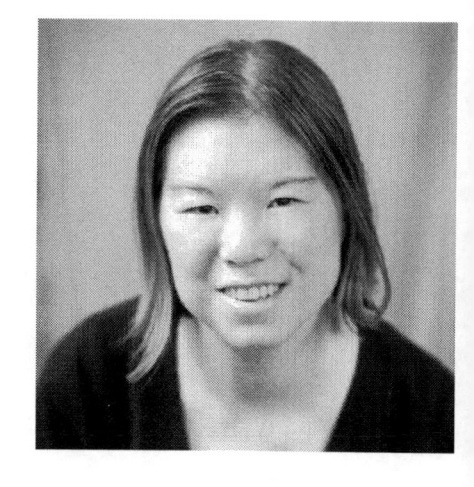

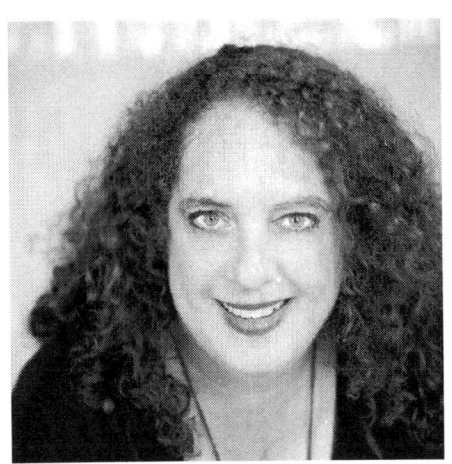

Rachel Orzoff
Everyday Rachel survives a severe traumatic brain injury, resulting from a fall down a flight of stairs. She does that in Minneapolis with the help of her amazing 11-year-old daughter.

Stevena Pen
Stevena was born in Minneapolis and raised in Saint Paul. While in the Marine Corps after high school, he has seen and done things no one could imagine. Follow, subscribe, and see some of the things he does and his journey though his recovery and success on YouTube: Penaloo

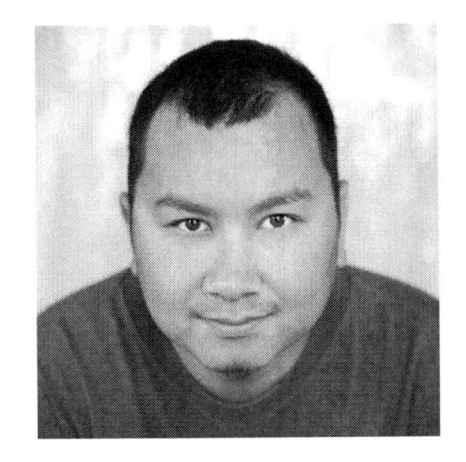

About the Author

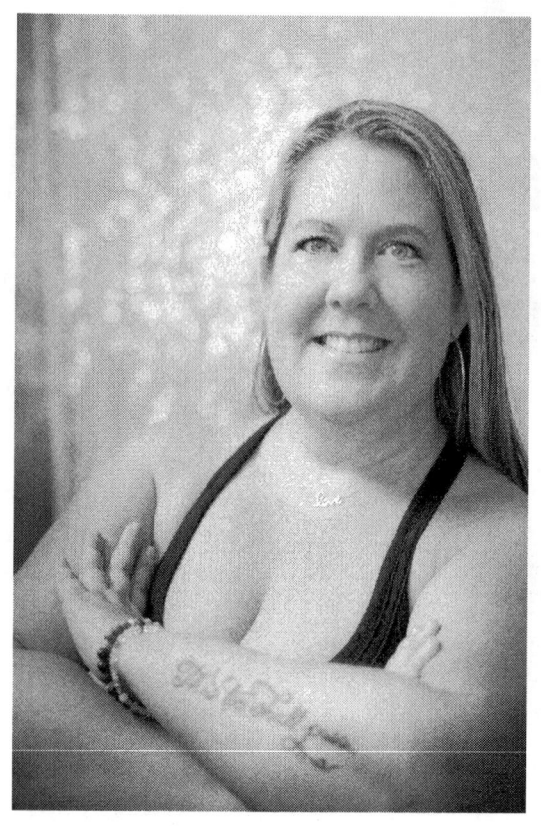

Amy Zellmer sustained a traumatic brain injury in February of 2014 after falling on the ice and landing full-force on the back of her skull. She is still recovering, and understanding the scope of her injury. She is an award-winning author, professional photographer, and creative business coach living in Saint Paul, Minnesota.

She is a frequent contributor to *The Huffington Post*, and produces a podcast series, "Faces of TBI," for survivors and their loved ones. She travels the country with her Yorkie, Pixxie, speaking to groups about this invisible injury that affects 2.5 million Americans each year.

Her first book *Life With a Traumatic Brain Injury: Finding the Road Back to Normal* received a silver medal in the Midwest Book Awards.

She is available for speaking at conferences and events, and may be reached through email: amyzellmertbi@gmail.com

She believes that the healing process begins with the telling of your story, releasing everything that you've been bottling up inside. TBI is an invisible disability that many don't understand. She wants to bring an awareness and understanding to the world, and hopes that people will have more compassion for those who look seemingly fine—but inside are struggling with memory or cognitive issues, such as she is.

Connect with Amy:
www.facesoftbi.com
www.facebook.com/facesoftbi
Twitter and Instagram: @amyzellmer

Made in the USA
Middletown, DE
10 December 2017